Dermatology

made easy

How to make the diagnosis

Dermatology
made easy:
How to make the diagnosis

Dr Thomas F. Poyner

FRCP (London & Glasgow) MRCGP

MAGISTER CONSULTING LTD

Dermatology made easy: How to make the diagnosis

by Dr Thomas F. Poyner FRCP (London & Glasgow) MRCGP

Published in the UK by
Magister Consulting Ltd
The Old Rectory
St. Mary's Road
Stone
Dartford
Kent DA9 9AS

Copyright © 2005 Magister Consulting Ltd
Printed in the UK by Nuffield Press, Oxfordshire

ISBN 1 873839 64 2

1. Infancy a new member in the family

Early rashes

Toxic erythema of the newborn

Presents within a few hours of birth

Red rash with small vesicles

Vesicles are sterile

Resolves in a few days

Transient neonatal pustulosis

Present at birth

Multiple pustules

No redness

Resolves in weeks without treatment

Milia

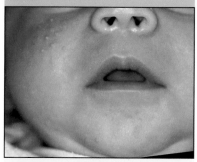

Due to ectodermal trapping

Small white cysts

Retention of keratin

Miliaria

Due to overheating

Small clear vesicles

Retention of eccrine sweat

Scaly rashes

Ichthyosis vulgaris

Autosomal dominant

Dry scaly skin

Flexural sparing

No erythema

Sex-linked ichthyosis

Due to deficiency of steroid sulphatase

More scaly and browner than ichthyosis vulgaris

No flexural sparing

No erythema

Xeroderma

Dry skin

Common with atopic eczema

Not as scaly as an ichthyosis

Keratosis pilaris

Rough horny plugs

Associations – atopic eczema and ichthyosis vulgaris

Often found on upper arms

More easily felt than seen

Nappy rash

Irritant dermatitis from urine and faeces

Erythema and scale in napkin area

Spares the folds

Satellite pustules suggest candida

Infantile seborrhoeic eczema

Starts at two to three months of age

Well baby

Scaly scalp and nappy rash

Can involve the flexures

Atopic eczema

Very common

Presents between six to 12 months

Starts on face

Localises to flexures

Itchy, scaly erythematous rash

Infant may be miserable

Scabies

Very itchy rash

Papules and eczematous patches

Pustules and burrows on palms and soles

Impetigo

Usual pathogen is *Staph. aureus*

Face is a common site

Yellow crusted lesions

Can blister

Acute blistering rash

Can be serious

See emergency dermatology section

Urticaria pigmentosa

Reddish brown macules

Urticates on rubbing

Naevi

Congenital naevi

Brown or black macules, or patches

Can develop hairs

Can present as giant naevi

Epidermal naevi

Warty linear lesions

Can undergo malignant change in later life

Café au lait

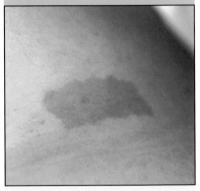

Common

Usually not significant

If present with axillary freckling, consider neurofibromatosis

Vascular lesions

Salmon patch or stork mark

Forehead, eyelids, nape of neck

Pink patches

Some resolve spontaneously

Strawberry mark

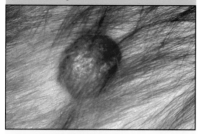

Superficial angioma

Develops in first weeks of life

Raised red lesion

Resolves spontaneously

Port wine stain

Head or neck

Deeper in colour than strawberry mark

Does not resolve with time

Exanthema
in infancy and childhood

Erythema infectiosum
(Fifth disease)

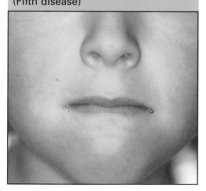

Erythema infectiosum
(Fifth disease) - continued

Erythrovirus B19

'Slapped cheek' appearance

Maculopapular rash

Can cause problems in pregnancy

Roseola

Herpes virus infection

Initial high fever

Morbilliform rash

Rash starts on trunk

Gianotti-Crosti syndrome

Various viruses

Symmetrical rash

More prominent on limbs

Red papular rash

Kawasaki disease

Cause unknown

Fever, lymphadenopathy

Strawberry tongue, cracked lips

Erythematous rash

Swelling of hands

Rash peels

Possible vascular complications

2. **Childhood** starting nursery and school

Atopic eczema / dermatitis

Itchy rash

In front of elbows, knees, ankles & wrists

Erythema, scale, lichenification & excoriations

Can become infected

Kaposi's varicelliform eruption
(eczema herpeticum)

Atopic eczema with herpes simplex

Extensive rash

Umbilicated vesicles and erythema

Scabies

Very itchy

Generalised papular rash

Burrows on backs of hands

Tinea capitis

Scaly rash in the scalp

Hair loss

Send samples for mycology

Head lice

Scalp irritation

Nits (eggs) on hairs

Lice on hairs

Excoriated scalp

Granuloma annulare

Annular lesions

Raised edge

Not scaly

Juvenile plantar dermatosis

Sweaty feet

Rash on soles

Eroded with pits

Juvenile spring eruption

Light induced, occurs in spring

Principally affects boys

Itchy papules on ears

Actinic prurigo

Light induced

Sun exposed sites

Very itchy papules and nodules

Related to PLE

Henoch-Schonlein purpura

Can be associated with a Strep. throat infection

Buttocks and legs

Vasculitis

Purpuric or urticated lesions

Warts

Due to HPV virus

Different types

Common warts

Back of hands

Around the nail beds

Rough papules

Verruca

Soles of the feet

Rough and hyperkeratotic lesions

Black dots in the lesion due to thrombosed capillaries

Filiform warts

Around nose, lips

Rough conical lesions

Molluscum contagiosum

Due to a DNA pox virus

Umbilicated papules

Flesh coloured

Can have a ring of eczema around lesions

3. Adolescence or where did we go wrong?!

Papular, pustular and vesicular rashes

Acne

Disease of pilosebaceous glands

Face and chest

Greasy skin

Blackheads and whiteheads

Papules and pustules

Occasional scarring

Severe acne

As above

Nodules – deeper inflamed lesions

Frequently scars

Types of acne scarring

Soft scars

Ice pick scars

Keloid scars

Herpes simplex virus

Facial lesions (can be other sites)

Triggered by sunlight

Vesicular lesions

Can become impetiginized

Scaly rashes

Pityriasis rosea

Viral aetiology?

Herald patch

Rash on trunk

Fir tree pattern

Macules with collarette of scale

Pityriasis lichenoides

Macules and papules and limbs

Acute form can resemble chickenpox

Lesions develop adherent scale

Tinea cruris

Usually affects males

Scaly rash in the groins

Spreading down the thighs

Spares the scrotum

Has a raised edge and central clearing

Co-existent tinea pedis

Tinea corporis

Red scaly annular rash

Raised edge

Central clearing

Confirm by mycology

Guttate psoriasis

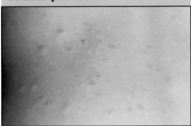

Triggers – streptococcal infection

Rash on the trunk

Multiple small scaly papules

'Raindrop' appearance

Polymorphic light eruption

2:1 ratio of females to males

Spring or early summer

Sun exposed sites

Comes on 24 hours after exposure

Itchy papules and plaques

Lasts a few days

Non scaly rashes

Vitiligo

Macular areas of depigmentation

No surface change

Face and hands

Tends to be symmetrical

More common in females

Can be associated with other auto-immune disease

Urticaria

Itchy wheals

Can be due to crab, shellfish, aspirin, penicillin

Associations – angioedema, dermatographism

Angioedema – swelling of the face, especially eyelids

Dermatographism – transient rash at sites of pressure

Erythema nodosum

Associations – Strep. throat, sarcoid and drugs

Lower shins

Hot, tender nodules

Erythema multiforme

Causes include herpes simplex, Mycoplasma

Symmetrical target / iris lesions

Can be bullous

Can have mucous membrane involvement

Itchy feet

Tinea pedis

Rash between the toes

Itchy and scaly

Can become more extensive (moccasin type)

Erythrasma

Due to a Corynebacterium

Sites axillae, groins, feet

Brown, scaly rash

Fluoresces under Wood's light

Differential diagnosis for tinea

4. Adults more work, less play!

Eczematous rashes (Dermatitis)

Atopic eczema/dermatitis

Often more severe than in children

Can present as for children

Can present as hand eczema

Irritant contact eczema/dermatitis

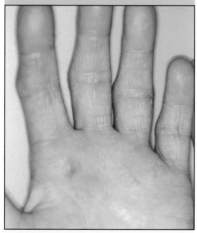

More common in those who have had atopic eczema

Often presents as hand eczema

Red scaly rash

Allergic contact eczema/ dermatitis

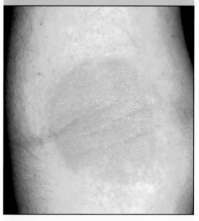

Common causes – nickel in a jean stud

Topical medications eg neomycin

Rash at site of contact

Discoid eczema

Red, coin-shaped palpable lesions

Covered in scale or crust

Tends to be symmetrical

Papulosquamous rashes
Scaly rashes with a well-defined edge

Psoriasis

Type one in adults

Tends to have a family history

Elbows, knees and lower back

Red plaques

Covered in silvery scale

Mycosis fungoides

Cutaneous T cell lymphoma

Scaly plaques

Gradually becoming more bizarre

Includes atrophy, telangiectasia and pigmentation

Erythroderma

Causes include psoriasis, eczema, lymphoma and drugs

Universal skin involvement

Red oedematous skin

Loss of heat, fluids and protein

Discoid LE

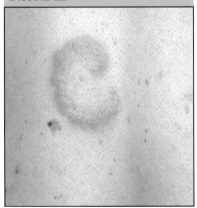

Discoid LE - continued

Face, scalp, chest and hands

Well-defined plaques

Follicular plugging

Telangiectasia and scarring

Aggravated by sunshine

Can cause scarring alopecia

Illustration: DLE simulating GA

Papulopustular rashes

Rosacea

More common in women

Worse in men

Facial rash, cruciate distribution

Erythema, papules and pustules

Nose – rhinophyma

Folliculitis

Usual pathogen – *Staph. aureus*

Common on limbs

Yellow pustules with surrounding erythema

Pseudomonas folliculitis

Associated with use of a Jacuzzi

Acute onset

Rash under area of the bathing costume

Multiple small pustules

Blistering rashes
Pemphigus

Intraepidermal blisters

Blisters that easily rupture

Circulating IgG antibodies

Dermatitis herpetiformis

Symmetrical itchy rash

Elbows, buttocks & knees

Vesicular lesions

Positive endomysial antibodies

Non scaly rashes
Alopecia areata

Associated with other autoimmune disease

Well defined areas of hair loss

Exclamation mark hairs

No scarring

Diffuse hair loss

Associated with iron deficiency and thyroid disease

No scarring

SLE

Female to male 8:1

'Butterfly' facial rash

Diffuse alopecia

Positive ANA, DNA

Multisystem disease

Malignancy
Melanoma

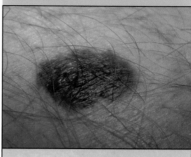

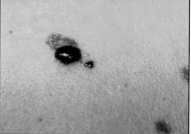

Female lower leg

Male back

Pigmented lesions

Superficial spreading or nodular

Recent change in size, shape or colour

Mixed colour, ulceration or inflammation

Kaposi's sarcoma

Can be a manifestation of HIV

Often on lower legs

Violaceous nodules

5. **Elderly skin** more play, less work!

Itchy scaly rashes

Skin Ageing

Chronological

Solar damage

Smoking (you have been warned!)

Genetic

Itchy dry skin

Often non-specific

May be due to soap and antiseptics

Need to exclude medical causes

Anaemia and lymphoma

Liver and renal disease

Seborrhoeic dermatitis

Scalp, face and chest

Nasolabial folds

Red scaly rash

Scale greasy (rather than silvery in psoriasis)

Asteatotic eczema

Dry skin

Lower legs

Crazy paving appearance

Varicose eczema

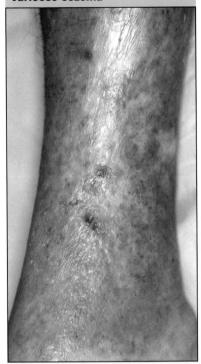

Gaiter area of the lower legs

Venous disease

Red scaly patches

Oedema, haemosiderin pigmentation

White areas of scarring (atrophy blanche)

Fibrosis

Lichen simplex

Very itchy rash

Nape of the neck & lower leg

Scaly plaques

Increased skin markings

Scabies

Common in nursing homes/
residential homes

Itchy rash

Burrows not always obvious

Psoriasis

Late onset – type 2

Tends to be mild

Less family history

Elbows, knees and lower back

Red, scaly plaques
(as psoriasis for other ages)

Drug Rashes

Toxic erythema

Psoriasiform

Blistering

Fixed drug eruptions

Erythroderma

Blisters
Pemphigoid

Sub-epidermal blisters

Erythematous base

Lack of oral involvement

Flexures
Interigo

Rash in flexures

Axillae, groins and
submammary folds

Red moist rash

Secondary infection common

Satellite pustules suggest candida

Light exposed areas
Actinic reticuloid

Rash on sun-exposed sites

Usually males

Eczematous plaques

Solar damage (solar elastosis)

Sun-exposed sites

Face, neck, forearms and hands

Yellowish skin and wrinkles

Pigmentation and stellate scars

Senile comedones

Sebaceous gland hyperplasia

Nails

Onychomycosis

Co-existent tinea pedis

Thickened, deformed nails

Need microscopy and culture

Differential diagnosis – psoriasis

Ulcers

Arterial ulcer

Foot or shin

Painful

Punched out, dry

Shiny, hairless skin

Reduced or absent peripheral pulses

History of claudication

Abnormal Doppler's

Venous ulcer

Lower leg

Superficial

Oedema, pigmentation

Eczema

Warm limb

Varicose veins

Diabetic ulcer

Over bony prominences

Painless

Deep

Lesions

Seborrhoeic warts
(Basal Cell Papilloma)

Face and trunk

Uniform brown lesions

Scaly, cribriform surface

Stuck-on appearance

Multiple, slow growing

Actinic keratoses

Sun-exposed sites

Small rough, scaly lesions

Slight risk of malignant change

Basal cell carcinomas

Face, neck & back

Nodule, cyst or plaque

Translucent, pearly surface

Raised edge

Telangiectasia

Can be pigmented

Very rarely spread

Bowen's disease

Lower leg or back of hand

Scaly patch

Risk of SCC

Squamous cell carcinoma

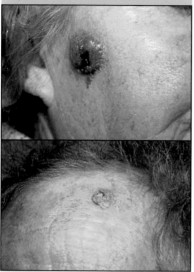

Lentigo maligna

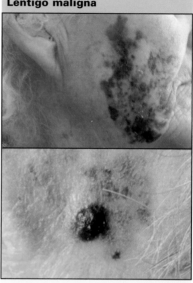

Sun-exposed sites

Nodule or non-healing ulcer

Slow growing

Keratoacanthoma

Sun-exposed site

Rapidly growing nodule

Central keratin plug

Face

Pigmented patch

Irregular margin and irregular pigmentation

Nodule can develop within the lesion, as illustrated

To Babs

and our physicians of the future -

Emma, Robin and Beth

About the Author

Thomas Poyner is a founder member, former chair and currently vice-chair of the Primary Care Dermatology Society. He is a full-time GP and was a clinical assistant and hospital practitioner in dermatology for 25 years. He is actively involved in teaching and education and is an honorary lecturer at Durham University, teaching undergraduates. He is also active in postgraduate education and his roles include acting as examiner for the diplomas in dermatology based at Cardiff, Glasgow and London. He takes the clinical skills and prescribing workshops for nurses at Teeside University.

Acknowledgements

Thanks also to Christine Dyer for proof reading and Dr Arthur Jackson and Dr A Carmichael for providing some of the slides.

Contents

Introduction

Patients in primary care frequently attend with a list of problems. Skin disease affects up to a third of the population and accounts for 15% of a GP's workload. Only 5% of those patients seen in primary care are referred to secondary care. This means that the average GP needs to be able to diagnose the majority of common skin diseases.

Many books are written to be used by those who do not need them. This book is designed for those in primary care and intermediate care who want to make the best diagnosis they can in the time available. It gives multiple points of entry to try to enable the user to make the same correct diagnosis. It has come out of years of experience and feedback from teaching GPs, medical students and nurses.

Part 1

Consultations

The first consultation

The patients usually consult because they either have a rash or a lesion. It is worth trying to ascertain how the patient sees the problem and what they hope to gain from the consultation. So often one gets lost in a quagmire of information and forgets exactly why the patient consulted in the first place.

There are various routes to diagnosis. These include the visual 'once-seen-never-forgotten' method. Another is taking a good history, performing a clinical examination and, where indicated, investigation. This book will help you to diagnose skin disease by a variety of techniques.

How to make a speedy diagnosis

There are those in a rush with a surgery to finish, the children to collect, a dinner to cook or the first tee beckoning! They want no frills dermatology. This book includes two sections: *The five ages of dermatology* inside the front cover and *What's likely from the signs and symptoms?* inside the back cover. These are designed for quick access, easy reference and can serve as an aide-memoire.

The five ages of dermatology – infancy, childhood, adolescence, adulthood and old age – are presented in a bullet point format and give you what is likely within that age group. However, any table has to be an over-simplification and many diseases can affect patients from cradle to grave!

Dermatology is a very visual subject and you can work at improving your visual recognition skills. When you have an interesting new case, have a read around it and consider keeping a picture of the rash or lesion. Gradually, you will build up a repertoire of skin diseases to which you can refer and you can develop the 'once-seen-never-forgotten' pattern recognition. When you are faced with a new skin complaint, your cerebral cortex will have a library of conscious and subconscious images that it can use to compare and contrast.

The logical pathway to diagnosis

This is the traditional didactic route involving taking a history, examining the patient and performing appropriate investigations.

History

Patients frequently complain that a rash is itchy, scaly or sore. They can be concerned that it's infectious, or are embarrassed by its appearance.

Key questions are:

- Where and when did it start?

- Where has it spread to?

- Has it changed?

- Does it vary in either severity or appearance?

- Any history or family history of skin disease?

- Any history or family history of atopy?

- What makes it better or worse?

- What bothers you most about it?

> **Tip:** do ask the patient what they think it is!

Previous history and family history

Family history is important as so many of the common skin diseases have a genetic component eg atopic eczema and psoriasis. It is worth asking for any history, or family history, of atopic conditions of eczema, asthma and psoriasis. If all the family have developed a new, itchy rash then scabies would be a distinct possibility.

Season variation, occupation and hobbies (see special section p. 116)

Many rashes such as psoriasis and acne usually improve with sunshine; however, a minority of patients become worse. There are certain individuals and occupations that are at increased risk of skin disease. It is worth inquiring about working abroad in hot, sunny climates. No history is complete without an inquiry into hobbies, pastimes and pets. It can throw up a lot of possibilities and does add some interest to the consultation!

What medications have been taken?

There are a few tips. Do ask what medications have been started recently, or obtained without prescription from the pharmacy or health food shop. Do look at the morphology of the rash as to a clue which drug could be responsible. Do consult more extensive texts for more drug possibilities. Do record drug interactions under sensitivities on the patient's computer record. This does stop the comment, 'That's funny, doctor. The last time you gave me those tablets they caused a similar rash.'

What has been applied?

Do ask about what's been tried either on prescription or from the pharmacy. Topical steroids can modify the appearance of the rash. With fungal infection, what you see is an immunological reaction to the fungus. Application of a topical steroid reduces this inflammation and produces the condition known as tinea incognito. Topical antibiotics can produce allergic contact dermatitis eg neomycin. Some topical antihistamines can cause allergic reactions.

Examination

If you're able to describe the rash, you are half-way there. Indeed, throw in a few Latin or Greek names and you might be taken for an expert! First, stand back and take a good look at the distribution – the rash is not going to disappear. Candidates in examinations often home in a few millimetres from the skin, perhaps looking for divine intervention!

It is worth looking from different angles and on different days. This is not so you can give yourself a second opinion, but more that rashes are evolving. With pityriasis rosea, for example, the initial herald patch can look very much like a fungal infection.

What sites are involved and distribution of rash

Certain rashes have a predilection for certain sites. A symmetrical distribution suggests an endogenous (constitutional) aetiology, ie something with a major genetic component. An asymmetrical rash favours an exogenous cause, ie something from the outside world, an infection perhaps, or a contact allergy.

Distribution

The distribution of a rash can help with diagnosis. Many diseases have a classical distribution:

- **Acne** – a rash on the face and chest with papules and pustules

- **Rosacea** – a papular facial rash with a cruciate distribution

- **Solar related condition** – a facial rash sparing behind ears and under chin

- **Psoriasis** – a scaly rash on the scalp, elbows, knees and lower back

- **Seborrhoeic eczema** – a scaly rash on the scalp, face, chest and flexures

- **Shingles** – follows a dermatomal distribution.

Morphology

Morphology describes the types of lesions in the rash. This is a chance to improve on the terms spot or pimple! For the purist these can be divided into primary lesions and secondary lesions. However, describing what you see seems to work in practice!

Primary lesion

Lesion	Description	Example
Macule	Small flat area <1cm	Eczema
Patch	Large flat area >1cm	Eczema
Papule	Small raised lesion < 1cm	Rosacea
Nodule	Large raised lesion > 1cm	Acne lesion
Plaque	Large flat topped lesion > 2cm	Psoriasis
Pustule	Containing purulent fluid	Acne lesion
Vesicle	Small fluid filled lesion < 0.5cm	Pompholyx
Bulla	Large fluid filled lesion > 0.5cm	Pemphigoid
Weal	Transient elevated area due to oedema	Urticaria

Secondary lesion

Lesion	Description	Example
Cyst	Fluid filled nodule with epithelial lining	Epidermoid cyst
Furuncle	Infection of hair follicle	
Carbuncle	Collection of furuncles	
Atrophy	Thinning of the skin	Steroid side effects
Fissuring	Cracks in the skin	Hand eczema
Sclerosis	Thickening of the skin	Lichen sclerosis
Maceration	Collection of moisture & debris	Intertrigo
Telangiectasia	Tiny dilated vessels	SLE, dermatomyositis

Surface (Go on, scratch it!)

- **Normal**

- **Scaly** – flaking

- **Lichenification** – thickening of the skin from scratching as in chronic eczema

- **Crust** – dried exudate

- **Warty** – rough

Secondary changes in the surface

- **Excoriation** – scratch mark

- **Erosion** – superficial loss of epidermis

- **Fissure** – split in the skin

- **Ulcer** – loss of epidermis and upper dermis

Colour

It is useful to define the colour of the rash, even though it may be obvious at the time. The redness of a rash is due to increased blood flow. Inflammation can result in both post inflammatory hypo and hyper pigmentation. Is it pink, red, or mauve? Psoriasis is either pink or red, whilst lichen planus tends to be mauve.

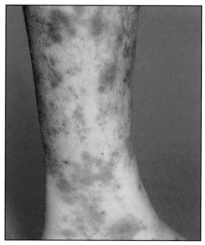

Lichen planus - note mauve colour

Primary lesion

Description	Explanation and examples
Erythema	Redness due to increased blood flow eg eczema
Erythroderma	Red all over
Leukoderma	White skin
Carotenaemia	Orange/yellow colour from fruits and vegetables
Purpura	Blood outside vessels
Petechiae	Small purpuric lesion
Ecchymosis	A bruise
Brown	Melanin eg lentigo
Green	Pseudomonas infection of nails

Border

It is worth observing to see if the border is regular or irregular. This can help distinguish benign from malignant lesions. A distinct edge between the rash and normal skin helps distinguish between psoriasis and eczema. A raised scaly edge is classical of ringworm and a raised smooth edge is present in granuloma annulare.

The shape of lesions

Term	Description	Example
Nummular	Coin like	Nummular eczema
Umbilicated	Central depression	Molluscum
Pedunculated	On a stalk	Papilloma
Verrucous	Warty	Wart on sole of foot

Configuration of lesions

- **Grouped** – lesions in one area

- **Discrete lesions** – separated by normal skin

- **Disseminated** – widespread discreet lesions

- **Linear** – in a line eg Koebner phenomenon

Palpate the skin (It won't bite!)

Is a lesion normal, soft, firm or hard? Do remove any crust from a lesion. Do feel purpura to see if it is palpable as in a vasculitis. Patches of morphea feel thickened whilst lichen sclerosis et atrophicus feels atrophic. Do stretch a suspected basal cell carcinoma as this makes the edge more easily seen.

Natural markings and creases

Artefactual rashes do not follow any biological line and do not follow the body's normal curves. Malignant lesions tend to destroy the skin's creases.

Look a little further afield

It is worth looking at other sites for clues: in the mouth at the buccal mucosa, for white patches in lichen planus. In psoriasis the nails may have pits or onycholysis (separation of the distal nail from its bed).

Whose sign!

It's nice to put a name to things, and dermatology is no exception:

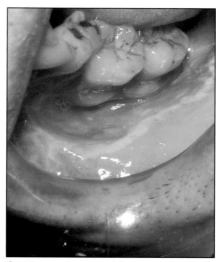

Oral lichen planus - white lace pattern

- **Darier's sign** is that a lesion in mastocytosis urticates or blisters on trauma.

- **Auspitz sign** is bleeding on scratching the last scale of psoriasis from a plaque

Terms for the honours' students!

Sometimes it's useful to try to understand what the dermatologist was viewing!

Term	Explanation
Arcuate	Curved
Follicular	Arising from hair follicles
Gyrate	Wavelike
Horn	Accumulation of abnormal keratin
Livedo	Blue colour
Reticulate	Netlike
Serpiginous	Snakelike

Tools (Boys like toys!)

It is worth examining a patient in a well-lit room. A magnifying glass is useful to look at finer detail with. A ruler is useful to measure lesions and a tape measure to record the circumference of a limb. A glass slide can be pressed over the skin (diascopy), purpura does not blanch and there is an 'apple jelly' appearance to lupus vulgaris. A torch can be used to inspect the mouth and give a short respite from conversation! Providing the practice nurses with a Doppler machine improves leg ulcer diagnosis and care.

Digital cameras enable you to take images and store them on the computer (a sign of wealth!). This, linked to the internet can be used in 'teledermatology' which might be thought of by some as 'phone a friend'!

A dermatoscope is a complicated bit of kit, used to help diagnose skin cancer. Those who go through the learning curve do find it useful.

Wood's light

This is ultraviolet light filtered through special glass. To shine a Wood's light on the skin in a darkened room takes only a few minutes and if nothing else gives you time to think. Having spent a large amount of money on an expensive Wood's light, its whereabouts in the surgery remains a mystery. Yet I am never without my hand-held lamp, courtesy of a pharmaceutical company. Wood's light is classically used when screening for cases of tinea capitis due to Microsporum infections. However, it has a multitude of uses.

Wood's light

Clinical Situation	Colour under Wood's light
Microsporum infections	Green-blue fluorescence
Pityriasis versicolor	Yellow fluorescence
Erythrasma	Coral pink fluorescence
Vitiligo	Delineates sites
Porphyria cutanea tarda	Urine gives pink fluorescence
Tuberose sclerosis	Ash leaf macules are more obvious

Investigation

Investigations can help to confirm a diagnosis. When a physician and surgeon examine a patient with abdominal pain they do a rectal examination and check the urine, so the GP faced with a scaly rash should perform mycology. In medicine, it's so often failure to do the simple test, rather than request the most complicated, that leads to problems. There are many complicated tests in dermatology to confuse the expert. When in doubt, ring your local laboratory for advice. They are often pleased to have a break from their microscopes and computers.

Bacterial swabs

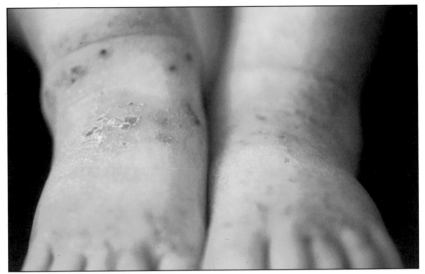

Infected atopic eczema

These are simple to take and worth considering when diagnosing infected eczema, impetigo, an acute paronychia and an infected ulcer.

Mycology

It is reasonable to diagnose tinea pedis on clinical grounds. However, at other sites tinea should be confirmed by mycology. One can take scrapings from any scaly rash eg tinea corporis and tinea cruris. From the scalp, one can take scrapings, hairs and samples using a non-sterile toothbrush. From the nails one can take clippings and sub ungula debris. Mycology samples are sent to the laboratory on black paper so they can be seen.

> **Tip:** If the diagnosis of a scaly rash is not obvious take samples for mycology.

Viral swabs

A herpetic lesion on the lip is quite easy to diagnose, but a similar lesion on a cheek, finger or buttock can be more difficult. Swabs can be taken for viral culture.

Blood tests

What do you do when faced with an itchy patient? The GP can screen for problems such as lymphoma, anaemia, liver and renal disease. Chronic urticaria is often idiopathic, but it is worth screening for thyroid disease. If the urticaria is associated with bruising and individual lesions are prolonged, then an urticarial vasculitis is a possibility and an ANA should be requested. If a rash is present on light exposed areas and worse on sun exposure then diseases such as SLE is a possibility. If there is scarring then porphyria should be excluded. If a patient has recurrent boils then anaemia, diabetes and reduced immunity are worth considering. In a case of purpura it is worth checking an FBC.

What's readily available?

Haematology

- FBC, ESR, WBC,

- CRP, Ferritin

Biochemistry

- U&E – RBS

- TFT

- LFTs – bile salts

- Testosterone, sex hormone binding globulin

- Prolactin – FSH, LH

- Porphyrins – blood, urine and faeces (special containers required)

Immunology

- ANA, DNA, ENA, Ro, La

- Endomysial antibodies

- Thyroid antibodies

- HIV (after counselling)

- RAST – test for allergen-specific IgE

- Indirect immunofluorescence tests for bullous diseases.

Appropriate investigations in clinical situations

Itch

- FBC, ESR, ferritin

- U&E, LFTS, TFT, RBS, CRP

- Endomysial antibodies

- CXR

Latex allergy

- RAST

Recurrent superficial infection eg boils

- FBC

- RBS, U&E

- Consider HIV testing

Urticaria

- TFT, LFTs
- FBC & ESR
- ANA and autoantibodies

Alopecia

- Ferritin
- Thyroid function
- Testosterone (females)

Hirsutism, PCOS

- U&E, RBS
- Testosterone, DHEAS
- FSH & LH, prolactin
- Abdominal ultrasound
- Morning & afternoon cortisol

Purpura

- FBC & ESR, coagulation studies
- ASO titre, autoantibodies
- LFTs, U&E
- Urine dipstick

Raynaud's phenomenon

- FBC & ESR

- Autoantibodies

- Cryoglobulins

- CXR for cervical ribs

Blisters

- Blood for endomysial antibodies

- Blood for indirect immunofluorescence

- Biopsy of blister for histology

- Biopsy for immunofluorescence

- Blood and urine for porphyrins

Patch testing

This is useful when investigating for allergic contact dermatitis. This is an immune response to contact with a potential allergen producing a delayed type 4 reaction. A potential allergen is applied to the skin and, if the patient is sensitised to it, they develop a rash approximately 48 hours later. Test substances are placed on inert small discs held in place on the patient's skin (usually the back) by adhesive dressings. After 48 hours the patch tests are removed and read with a further reading being repeated after 96 hours from slower reactions. A positive test produces an area of palpable erythema.

The test substance is made up in a solid base. There is a European standard battery and other batteries for certain situations and occupations. Patch testing is a combination of an art and a science. Some substances can produce both immediate and delayed reactions and others can irritate. One may have a positive result, but one has to decide, 'Is it clinically relevant?'

Prick tests

Prick tests are often confused with patch tests. Prick tests are looking for an immediate reaction to a test substance. This test is not very popular in dermatology and is more suited to those involved in diagnosing 'allergy'. Some dermatologists do prick tests for latex; but there is the risk of producing anaphylaxis. If latex allergy is suspected, a RAST test is simpler and safer in primary care.

Photo testing

There are various ways of testing for light related problems. Photo testing is done in secondary care to investigate possible photosensitivity to medicines. Photo provocation tests are used to test for rashes, such as polymorphic light eruption. Photo patch testing is used in testing for a photocontact allergy.

Skin biopsy

In less cerebral areas of medicine there is a maxim of 'when in doubt cut it out'! However, in dermatology, before dashing to the scalpel, think long and hard about what is going to be gained by taking a biopsy. Any lesion is best treated by excision biopsy rather than incisional biopsy. Always send any material for histology. Do give plenty of information with the specimen. Only do a biopsy if you are ready and able to act on the result.

Types of biopsy

There are various types of biopsy. These include:

- Incisional

- Excisional

- Punch

- Shave

- Curettage and cautery

- Snip

Before the blade strikes!

Before you embark on your career as a dermatological surgeon think:

Why are you doing a biopsy?

Are you the most appropriate person?

How will it take you forward?

What will you do with the result?

A shave excision can be used for seborrhoeic warts. For a rash, one would be doing a punch biopsy and the edge of a rash is often the most active area. Samples can be sent for histology and immunofluorescence (especially blistering rashes). For a case of suspected mycosis fungoides, multiple biopsies are required from different sites.

Applied anatomy of the skin

The word anatomy turns most physicians off. However, a little revision of the applied anatomy can be quite useful. The skin is composed of the epidermis, dermis and adipose tissue.

Surface change in a rash such as scale suggests a disease involving the epidermis eg eczema and psoriasis. If the disease is deeper in the skin eg granuloma annulare, then there is no scale. Vascular dilation produces redness eg rosacea and eczema. Blood outside vessels causes purpura.

The skin has various glands, including pilosebaceous glands and apocrine glands. Pilosebaceous glands are plentiful on the face and chest.

Obstruction of them occurs in acne producing blackheads and whiteheads. Inflamed lesions derived from sebaceous glands eg papules and pustules are found in acne and rosacea.

The blisters in the immunobullous diseases occur at different levels in the skin. Those of pemphigus are intraepidermal whilst in pemphigoid they are deeper, being subepidermal.

> **Tip:** *Because the blister of pemphigus is superficial, it is soon lost.*

Part 2

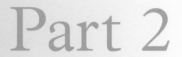

Overview

of some of

the common

rashes and

problems

Whilst there are over 3,000 dermatological conditions one could encounter, just a few diseases dominate the majority of the consultations in primary care.

Acne

Acne is a disease of the pilosebaceous glands. These are plentiful on the face and chest and absent from the hands and feet. The physiological surge of androgens at puberty affects these glands with increased sebum production and duct obstruction. The increased sebum production is associated with a greasy skin. Virtually all teenagers have some acne, but the severity reflects the individual's sebaceous glands' sensitivity to androgens. This is partly genetic but, sadly, for some, taking anabolic steroids plays a part. Anything that increases duct obstruction such as oils and greases can aggravate acne.

Acne has non-inflamed lesions, open comedones (whiteheads) and closed comedones (blackheads). Inflammatory lesions develop with

Acne - papules and pustules

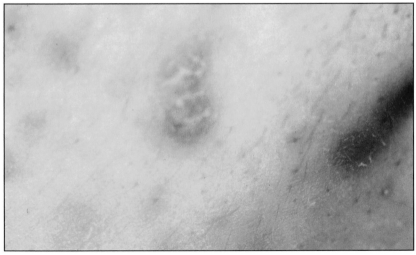

increasing numbers of *P. acnes* in the obstructed ducts. There are papules, pustules and deeper larger lesions (nodules). Acne can go on to scar and scarring is usually, but not exclusively, associated with severe acne. Types of scarring include atrophic, ice pick and keloid.

Acne scarring

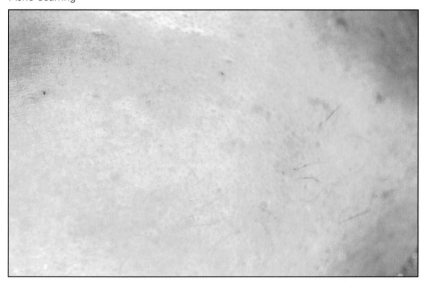

It is worth trying to grade acne as mild, moderate or severe. The severity of rash on the face and back can be quite different between face and chest, so it is worth viewing both sites. Both acne and rosacea have papules and pustules. Acne can be distinguished from rosacea as acne does have blackheads and whiteheads and rosacea does not. Acne is associated with a greasy skin (seborrhoea), rosacea is not.

Eczema (dermatitis)

The term eczema and dermatitis are synonymous and are used to describe inflammation of the skin. Dermatitis has in the past been reserved for conditions thought to be due to environmental factors eg those associated with an occupation.

Eczema with fissure

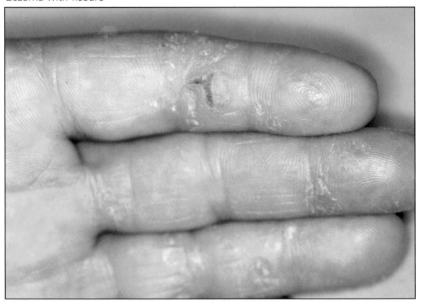

Eczema may be acute with erythema, vesiculation and weeping. Alternatively, the eczema can be chronic with scale, fissures and lichen-ification. Frequently, what one sees in clinical practice is a combination of acute eczematous changes on a chronic background.

There are various ways of trying to classify eczema and these include causation, appearance, site and age of onset. Some patients fit neatly into one group, whilst for others the aetiology of their rash tends to be multi-factorial.

When trying to come to an accurate diagnosis, factors worth considering include age at onset, past medical history, family history, occupational history, site and appearance of the rash.

Atopic eczema/dermatitis

Atopic eczema - hand involvement

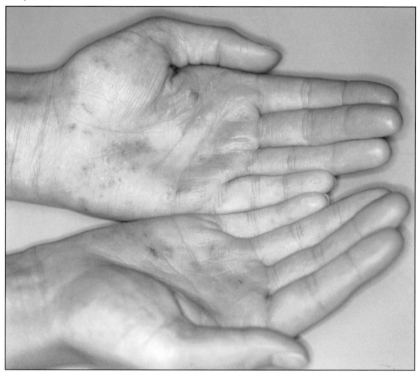

Atopic eczema affects between 15 to 20 per cent of school children and the prevalence is increasing. Sixty per cent of those affected develop the rash in the first year of life. Eighty per cent of cases classed are mild and, for 60 per cent, the rash clears at adolescence. Atopic eczema has a relapsing course with flares. Two to three per cent of adults have atopic eczema and their rash tends to be worse than that of children. It either affects the same sites as children, or presents as hand eczema.

Hand eczema - erythema, scale and fissures

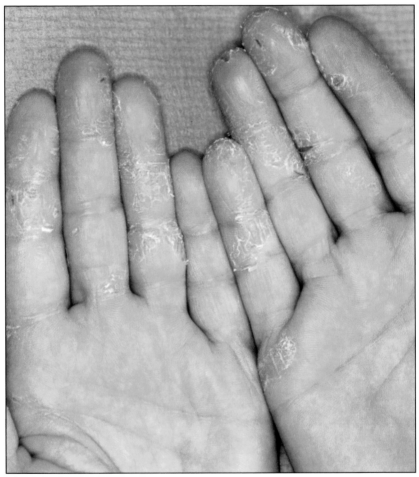

Atopic eczema is one of the atopic conditions and is associated with the other atopic conditions of asthma and hay fever. Seventy to 80 per cent have a family history and their rash is probably a combination of 50 per cent genetic susceptibility and 50 per cent environmental factors. These factors include house dust mites and hard water. Atopic eczema is more prevalent in smaller families and is associated with affluence. The role of diet is somewhat controversial.

Atopic eczema starts in infancy with a rather non-specific facial eruption with variable involvement of the trunk. The child goes on to develop a symmetrical red rash in the skin creases, with patches affecting the folds in front of elbows and behind the knees. The rash can affect the wrists and ankles. In the acute phase the rash can have vesicles, whilst in the chronic phase there is lichenification due to the scratching.

Keratosis pilaris - easier to feel than see

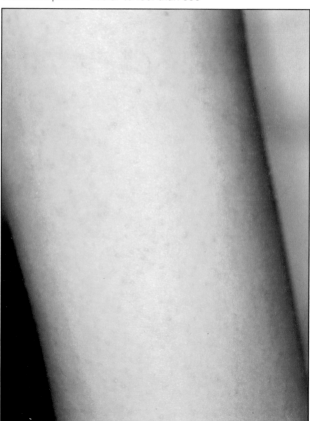

There is a background of a generally dry skin. Keratosis pilaris is found in both atopic eczema and ichthyosis vulgaris. These are small rough papules found on the upper arms that are more easily felt than seen.

Ichthyosis - dry skin with scale

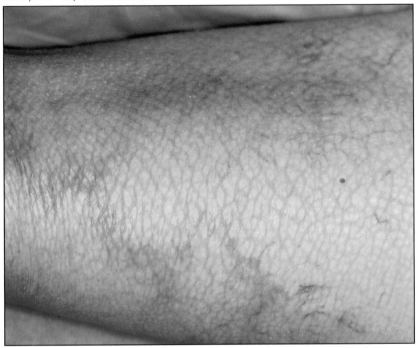

There is often facial pallor and atopic eczema is associated with pityriasis alba, with pale scaly patches on the child's face. In atopic eczema there can be both hyperpigmentation and hypopigmentation, with reticulate pigmentation on the neck. In some children from certain ethnic groups (Asian and Afro-Caribbean) the rash tends to be more extensor than flexor.

Atopic eczema is itchy and the scratching produces excoriations. This, combined with the reduced barrier function of the atopic skin leads to secondary infection. The secondary infection causes a further deterioration in the eczema. A sudden deterioration of eczema should alert one to the possibility of secondary infection. Other signs of infection include weeping and pustulation.

Herpes simplex infection on a background of active atopic eczema can cause a devastating rash of eczema herpeticum (extensive vesicles of an erythematous background).

Eczema herpeticum - atopic eczema and herpes simplex

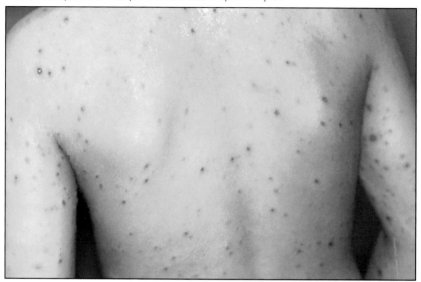

Contact dermatitis/eczema

There are two main types of contact dermatitis – irritant and allergic.

Irritant contact dermatitis/eczema

This is due to skin coming into contact with irritants and will depend on the individual's susceptibility, the strength of the irritant and the frequency and duration of exposure to the irritant. Any patient can develop an irritant eczema, although those with atopic eczema have a skin with reduced barrier function and are therefore more susceptible.

Certain occupations are more prone to irritant eczema (see occupational dermatology section on page 119). Weak irritants would be soaps, detergents and soluble oils, whilst stronger irritants are bleaches, caustics and petroleum.

The hands are the first part of the body that usually come into contact with an irritant. An itchy red rash develops in the webs between the fingers, then spreads to involve the rest of the hands. Nappy rash is an irritant eczema and it affects the convex areas with sparing of the flexures in between the folds of skin.

Contact dermatitis - nickel jean stud

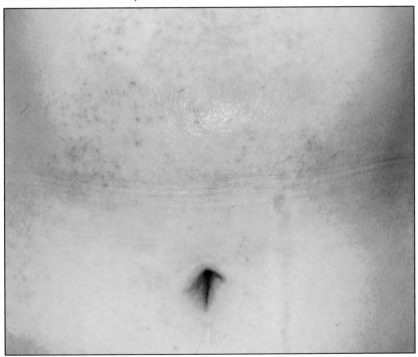

Allergic contact dermatitis/eczema

This is usually due to a delayed reaction (type four) to a substance. Before there can be an allergic reaction there has to be some initial sensitisation. Then, on subsequent contact, a rash develops, usually one to three days later.

Contact dermatitis - rubber glove

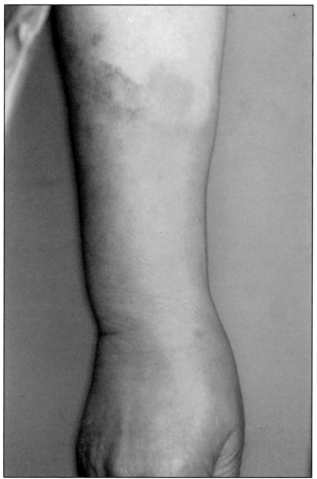

Common reactions are a rash on the abdomen from nickel in a jean stud, a rash in the scalp and hairline from paraphenylendiamine in hair dyes and on the hands from rubber gloves. If one suspects an allergic contact dermatitis then the patient should be referred for patch testing.

A repeated application test can be performed by a daily application of a small amount of the test substance (eg to the elbow) for a short period and observing for a reaction. This simple test can be done in primary care, especially if one suspects the patient's own medication may be to blame.

Common allergen	Common source
Antihistamines	Topical medication
Chromate	Cement and leather
Colophony	Sticking plasters
Epoxy resins	Adhesives
Fragrances	Perfumes, cosmetics
Lanolin	Topical medication
Local anaesthetics	Creams
Neomycin	Topical antibiotics
Nickel	Jewellery, jean studs
Paraphenylendiamine	Hair dyes, shoes
Preservatives	Cosmetics, creams
Primula	Plants
Rubber chemicals	Boots, gloves, shoes and tyres

Seborrhoeic dermatitis/eczema

This affects seborrhoeic areas, but is not associated with increased sebum production. It is, however, associated with increased colonisation with the Pityrosporum yeast. Severe adult seborrhoeic dermatitis can be associated with HIV.

Seborrhoeic dermatitis is common and, in its mildest form, presents as dandruff. As the rash becomes more severe, greasy scale forms in the scalp. The face can be involved with a scaly erythematous rash in the nasolabial folds, eyebrows and ears. Seborrhoeic dermatitis is itchy. It can affect the chest presenting with a petaloid rash. There can be involvement of the flexures with secondary infection. Infantile seborrhoeic eczema presents earlier than atopic eczema and with a well child. There can be extensive scalp and napkin area involvement.

Infantile seborrhoeic eczema - scaly scalp, no hair loss

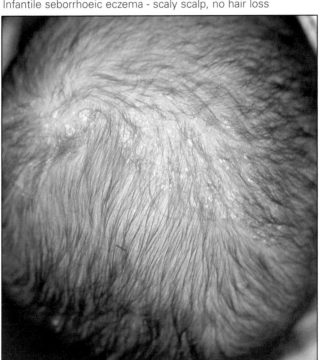

> **Tip:** If an infant has cradle cap and nappy rash consider infantile seborrhoeic dermatitis.

Discoid eczema

Discoid eczema (nummular eczema) presents with very itchy coin shaped lesions on the limbs. The lesions can be vesicular, crusted or covered in scale. They can be difficult to distinguish from psoriasis. The surface is frequently secondarily infected, which is unusual with psoriasis.

Discoid eczema - coined shaped lesions

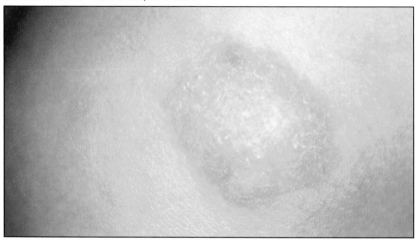

Other eczemas

For pompholyx and hyperkeratotic hand eczema, see sections on hands and feet (page 103). For asteatotic eczema and varicose eczema, see the section on rashes on the lower legs (page 97).

Psoriasis

Patients often ask why they have got psoriasis. We do not have all the answers, but what is known is that there is frequently a family history and, for some, there are certain aggravating factors. These include infection, trauma, medications eg beta blockers and antimalarials. Many patients report that stress aggravates their psoriasis. Many find their psoriasis improves with sunlight but, in a minority, it gets worse. Alcohol can be a factor and tobacco smoking is associated with localised pustular psoriasis.

Psoriasis - well defined scaly plaques

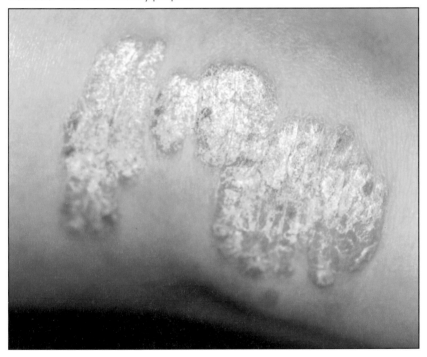

Psoriasis presents as well defined erythematous scaly plaques. Classical sites are the scalp, lower back, elbows and knees. The silvery scale and the well defined edge help to distinguish psoriasis from eczema. The rash can be itchy and there can be nail involvement. The nails are thickened, deformed, with pits and separation of the distal nail from its bed (onycholysis). Psoriasis can form in scars and this is known as the Koebner phenomenon. Psoriatic arthritis can present in many ways, and in some resembles rheumatoid disease.

Guttate psoriasis - small scaly lesions

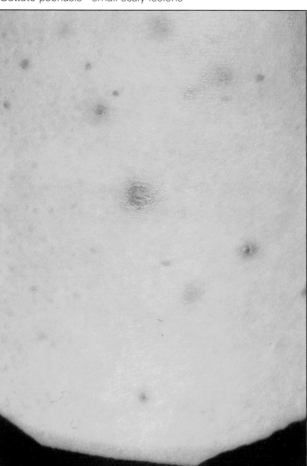

Guttate psoriasis classically presents in a young person with a generalised rash that has a raindrop appearance. It is frequently preceded by a strep-tococcal sore throat. Localised pustular psoriasis presents in middle-aged female smokers. Their palms and soles are red with sterile reddish-brown pustules.

Urticaria

Urticaria (hives) presents with intensely itchy wheals. Acute urticaria may be due to strawberries, crab, aspirin or shellfish. Chronic urticaria is when the disease has been going on beyond six weeks. Most cases of chronic urticaria are classified as idiopathic, although some may be autoimmune. Urticaria can be associated with angioedema, with facial swelling and even laryngeal oedema.

Urticaria - transient itchy wheals

It is worth asking about a past history of atopy, and thyroid function should be checked as thyroid disease can aggravate urticaria. Other tests worth considering are a FBC, ESR, LFTs and autoimmune screen. Medication such as aspirin, ACE inhibitors and non-steroidal anti-inflammatory drugs can aggravate urticaria. Other types of urticaria include the physical urticarias. Urticaria can be precipitated by heat, cold, pressure and water. Certain food additives such as tartrazine and azo dyes can aggravate it. In cholinergic urticaria there is an urticarial rash consisting of multiple tiny wheals appearing after exercise or stress.

Dermographism presents as whealing under pressure sites eg under straps. It can be elicited by stroking the skin. Pressure urticaria is different, in that there is a delay between the pressure stimulus and the rash.

If the individual wheals are prolonged (more than 24 hours) and there is bruising and arthralgia, then there may be an urticarial vasculitis and an ANA should be requested. Latex allergy can produce both immediate and delayed responses. It can cause severe reactions including anaphylaxis. Health workers are at increased risk. If there is any doubt it is worth doing a RAST test.

Common Superficial Infections

Bacterial infections

One can divide bacterial infections by their site in the skin:

- **epidermis (full thickness)** – ecthyma

- **upper dermis** – erysipelas

- **lower dermis** – cellulitis

- **fascia** – necrotising fasciitis
  (see emergency dermatology on page 124)

Staphylococcal infections (occasionally Streptococcal) tend to produce localised lesions. These infections include impetigo, folliculitis, boils and ecthyma (a superficial infection with ulceration and a crust).

Streptococcal infections (occasionally Staphylococci) tend to produce areas of infection rather than localised lesions. These include erysipelas and cellulitis. The former usually presents as a red, warm oedematous area on the face and the latter as a hot swollen leg. The patient with these infections frequently is generally unwell, with a fever and malaise.

Fungal infections

Fungal infections are often due to either yeasts or dermatophytes. Candida, a yeast, can cause oral thrush, a vulvovaginitis, secondary infection of intertrigo and a chronic paronychia. The yeast Malassezia furfur causes pityriasis versicolor and is also implicated in adult seborrhoeic dermatitis.

Candida - note satellite pustules

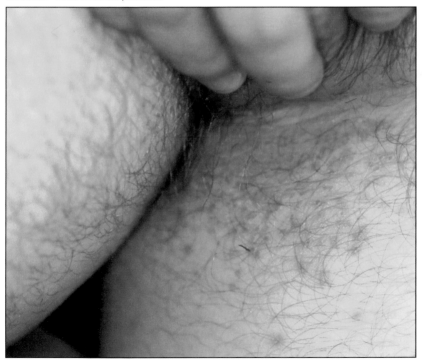

The dermatophytes are branching fungi. The most common infection is tinea pedis (athlete's foot). This presents as an itchy rash on the feet. Involvement usually starts between the fourth and fifth toes and the infection can spread to the toenails. Tinea can also spread to the groin.

Tinea pedis - itchy scaly rash

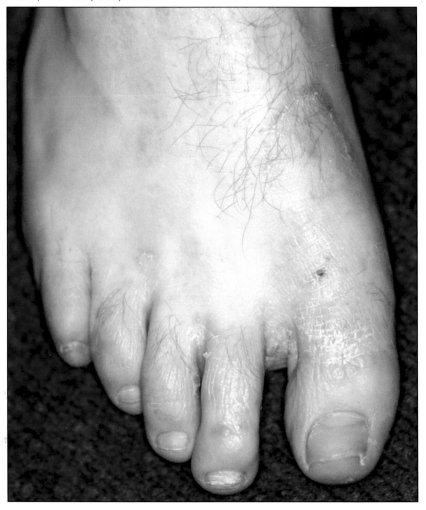

Tinea cruris appears as a red scaly rash with an active edge. There is scrotal sparing. Tinea corporis presents as red scaly coin-shaped lesions. Tinea on the neck and face can be quite pustular and be due to cattle ringworm. Scalp ringworm (tinea capitis) presents as scaly areas in the scalp with hair loss.

Viral infections

Herpes simplex can affect the lips and genitalia, presenting with a recurrent painful vesicular eruption. Herpes zoster (shingles) presents with a vesicular rash on an erythematous base that follows a dermatomal distribution. There is usually a severe prodromal pain.

Herpes zoster exhibiting dermatomal distribution

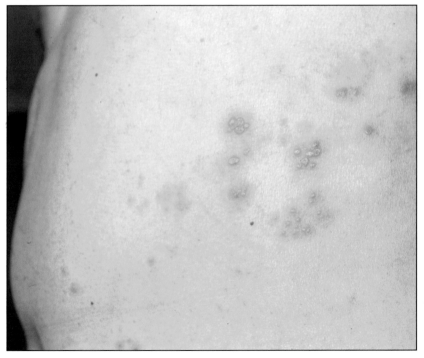

Scabies

Scabies is very itchy, with the itch being worse at night. Several family members are frequently affected. The rash presents as papular eczematous patches. Burrows can be difficult to find and it is worth looking in the finger webs. Infants can have vesicles on the soles of the feet. Penile lesions are diagnostic in the male. Inappropriate prescribing of topical steroids can reduce the inflammation. Those with reduced immunity can present with crusted scabies. Scabies is especially a problem for certain communities. These include those in residential and nursing homes, and asylum seekers.

Drug Rashes

You name it and a drug can cause it! Some drug rashes are idiosyncratic, whilst others are dose related. Drugs can both produce and aggravate

Toxic erythema - often due to medication

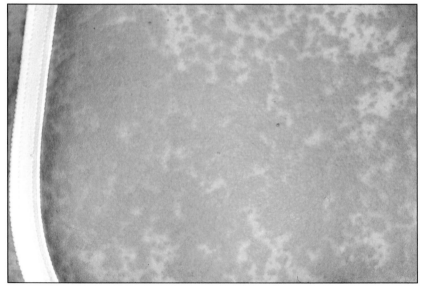

rashes eg aspirin and urticaria. Other medications, especially antibiotics, can produce a toxic erythema (red blotchy rash). Some drugs can interact with light to produce a rash eg doxycycline. Fixed drug eruptions occur at the same site every time the drug is taken and a classical fixed drug eruption would be a scaly patch on a limb after taking a laxative.

Type of rash	Example of drugs
Urticaria	Aspirin, penicillin and sulphonamides
Acneform	Lithium, steroids, phenytoin
Blisters	ACE inhibitors, NSAI, diuretics
Eczematous	Penicillin, sulphonamides, thiazides
Erythema nodosum	Contraceptives, gold, sulphonamides
Erythema multiforme	Penicillin, sulphonamides, thiazides
Exfoliative dermatitis	Anti-malarial, anticonvulsants, gold
Fixed drug eruption	Laxative, sulphonamides, tetracycline
Lichenoid	ACE inhibitors, carbamazepine, penicillamine
Light related	Bendrofluazide, tetracyclines, sulphonamides
Lupus-like	Captopril, carbamazepine, hydralazine
Morbilliform	Antibiotics, barbiturates, phenothiazines
Vasculitis	Allopurinol, antibiotics, thiazides

Part 3

What is likely

at each site

Certain diseases are more common at certain sites and this can be used as an aid to diagnosis.

Face and neck

The face is very important as it is a visible site. Common problems are a spotty, red face and a scaly, red face.

The Spotty red face

Acne (see common rashes, page tbc)

Acne affects the face, chest and back. There is a greasy skin. There are non-inflamed lesions from obstruction of the pilosebaceous glands. These are blackheads and whiteheads. There are also inflammatory lesions (papules and pustules). In more severe acne there can be nodules. Scarring is more common with severe acne.

Mild acne - few papules and pustules

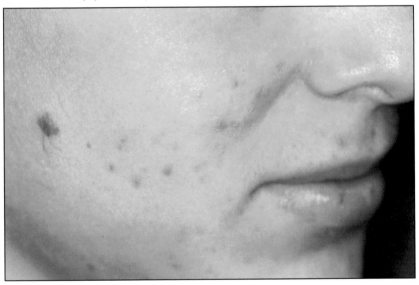

Rosacea

Rosacea is more common in middle-aged females, although males have more complications. There is a facial rash in a cruciate distribution. There are inflammatory lesions of papules and pustules on a background of erythema. In rosacea there are no blackheads or whiteheads. Patients with rosacea frequently complain of flushing that may be related to foods. A rhinophyma (bulbous nose) is more common in men. Rosacea can cause ophthalmic problems.

Rosacea - red rash, cruciate distribution

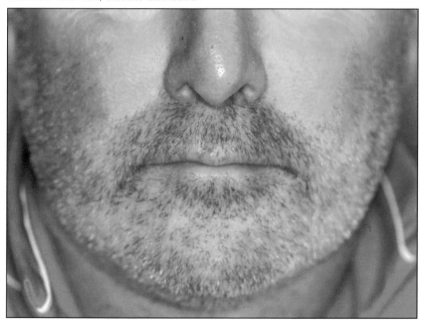

Tip: *Rosacea, unlike acne, does not have comedones, nor is there increased sebum production.*

Perioral dermatitis

This usually presents in young women with a rash around the mouth consisting of papules and pustules. This acneform rash may be induced by inappropriate use of topical steroids.

Perioral dermatitis - papules, pustules around the mouth

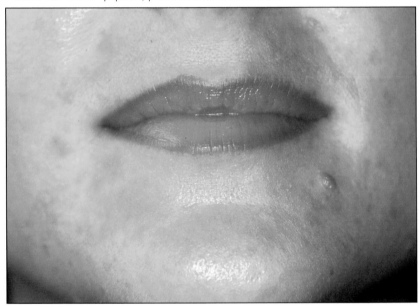

Angioedema

Facial swelling that can be associated with urticaria (wheals) and difficulty with breathing. It is worth inquiring if there is any association to foods or medicines such as shellfish, strawberries, nuts and penicillin.

Superficial skin infections of the face

The face is prone to bacterial, fungal and viral infections.

Impetigo

Impetigo is common on the face and can be primary or secondary to herpes simplex lesion (cold sore). It presents as yellow crusted lesions and is usually due to *Staph. aureus*.

Impetigo - yellow crusted lesions

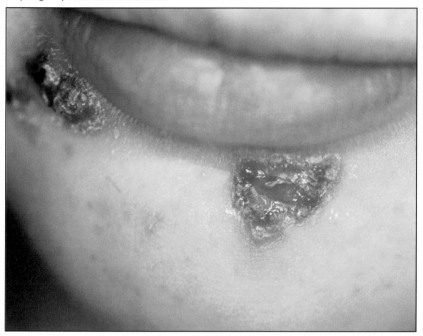

Folliculitis

A folliculitis of the face often presents as a widespread pustular eruption of the beard area (sycosis barbae). Ingrowing facial hairs can produce a similar appearance (pseudo sycosis barbae).

Folliculitis - infected hair follicles

Erysipelas (see emergency dermatology, page 124)

The patient is unwell with a warm expanding patch with a demarcation of abnormal skin. This is usually due to a streptococcal infection.

Herpes simplex

Herpes simplex on the face and lips presents as painful vesicular lesions that can go on and become impetiginized. Sunlight and menstruation can provoke recurrent attacks. The first symptom is tingling at the affected site.

Herpes simplex - vesicular lesions

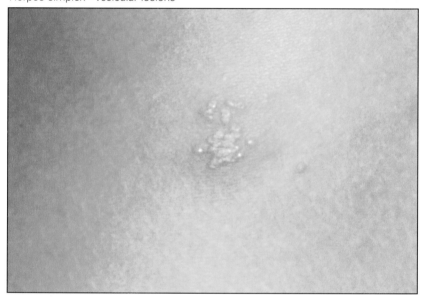

Spotty faces

Milia

- Contain keratin
- Face and genitalia
- Small firm cyst
- White or cream colour

Syringomas

- Cheeks
- Small smooth white papules

Dermatosis papulosa nigra

- Found in Afro-Caribbeans
- Related to seborrhoeic warts
- Facial lesions
- Multiple small black papules

Scaly red face

Seborrhoeic dermatitis

Seborrhoeic dermatitis presents as an itchy scaly erythematous rash affecting the face and scalp. Facial involvement includes the nasolabial folds, eyebrows and ears. Otitis externa is not uncommon. The scale of seborrhoeic dermatitis tends to be greasy compared with the silvery scale of psoriasis. Seborrhoeic dermatitis can involve the flexures, but unlike psoriasis does not produce any nail involvement.

The scale of seborrhoeic dermatitis helps distinguish it from rosacea.

Discoid lupus erythematosus tends to scar, whilst seborrhoeic eczema does not. Seborrhoeic dermatitis in the flexures is frequently secondarily infected by candida and Staph. aureus.

Atopic eczema

Atopic eczema frequently affects the face, although it is usually mild. There is dryness of the skin, frequently facial pallor and eyelid involvement. Pityriasis alba is related to atopic eczema. It presents as dry, scaly, erythematous patches on the cheeks of children.

Pityriasis alba - pale cheeks

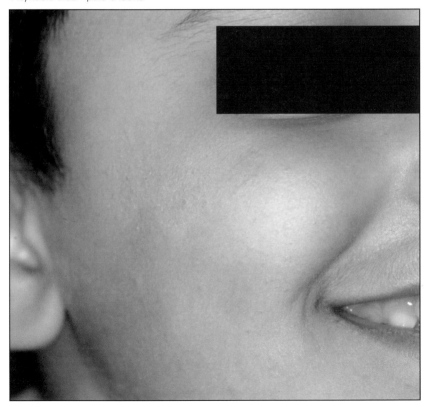

Allergic contact dermatitis

Presented with any new case of facial eczema one should consider, 'Could this be a contact allergic eczema?' The eyelids can be affected by allergy to nail varnish, and the neck to perfumes. The diagnosis is confirmed by patch testing. An airborne contact dermatitis affects exposed sites such as the face and neck. It does not spare the skin creases as does a photosensitivity rash.

Photosensitivity rashes

Photosensitivity rashes affect exposed sites such as the face, neck and arms. There is sparing under the hair line, behind the ears and under the chin. There is a sharp demarcation to the rash at the neckline. It is worth asking about medication that could be implicated eg tetracyclines and bendrofluazide. It is also worth screening for SLE by asking for an ANA and requesting blood and urine porphyrins.

Psoriasis

Psoriasis can involve the face and, when it does, it can resemble seborrhoeic eczema. However, the diagnosis of psoriasis is aided by seeing hairline involvement with a well demarcated edge, psoriatic plaques at other sites and nail involvement.

Tinea faciale

A fungal facial infection is usually due to animal ringworm and therefore is frequently found in farming communities. There is a very angry rash, with pustules and nodules. Secondary bacterial infection is common and can lead to diagnostic difficulty.

Collagen diseases

SLE

- 'Butterfly' facial rash
- Light aggravated
- Multi system involvement
- Positive immunology

Discoid lupus erythematosus

- Well-defined plaques
- Adherent scale
- Changes in pigmentation
- Scarring
- Look for scalp involvement

Subacute cutaneous LE

- Face or chest
- Annular or papulosquamous
- 50 per cent have systemic problems

Dermatomyositis

- Mauve (heliotrope) rash around the eyes
- Backs of the hands violaceous papules (Gottron's papules)
- Nail fold changes of telangiectasia and infarcts.

Tip: Patients with the butterfly rash of systemic lupus are unwell, compared to those with rosacea.

Sarcoid and TB on the face

Lupus pernio

- Sarcoid affects nose and ears
- Involved sites are deep purplish colour

Lupus vulgaris

- TB of skin
- Reddish brown plaques
- Variable scale
- Diascopy – apple jelly nodules

Red nodular facial rashes

Granuloma faciale

- Vasculitis
- Nodules on the face
- Red-brown in colour

Jessner's lymphocytic infiltrate

- Benign lymphocytic infiltrate
- Face and chest
- Purple nodular lesions

Sweet's Syndrome

- Fever
- Rash on limbs or face
- Plum coloured plaques

The lips

The lips can be a site for both contact irritant and allergic dermatitis. They are also a favourite site for herpes simplex and solar damage. Actinic cheilitis presents with an inflamed scaly lower lip, with loss of vermilion border. Angular cheilitis occurs in iron deficiency.

Scalp and hair

Consultations and hair biology

Patients are usually bothered because they either have too little or too much hair. Hair problems can be localised or generalised. Hair undergoes a growing phase (anagen), a resting phase (telogen) and a shedding phase (catagen).

When dealing with scalp problems important points are:

- Increased hair shedding

- Generalised or localised alopecia (hair loss)

- Scaling

- Scarring

- Any rash at other sites

- A family history of hair problems

Scaly scalps with no hair loss

Scaly scalps are usually due to seborrhoeic dermatitis, psoriasis, or fungal infections. With seborrhoeic eczema the scale is rather greasy, whilst in psoriasis it is silvery. The rash of psoriasis tends to extend below the hairline and has a well defined edge. Hair loss is unusual with both psoriasis and seborrhoeic dermatitis, but common in tinea capitis. In tinea amiantacea there is scale along the hairs; this can be due to either psoriasis or eczema. An acute eczematous reaction in the scalp can result from allergic reactions to hair dyes.

Scalp psoriasis - scaly red rash

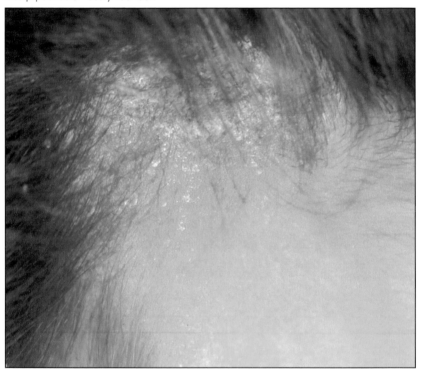

Pediculosis capitis (head lice)

Thankfully, most cases of head lice are more often diagnosed by the patient or relatives. Head lice cause scalp irritation and this may be severe enough to cause excoriations and even secondary infection. Nits (eggs) and live lice are seen on the hairs. The excoriations and impetiginized rash are more often on the nape of the neck.

Scaly scalps with hair loss

If there is scale and hair loss then one should be suspicious of tinea capitis. Ringworm commonly, but not exclusively, affects children. The infection can be contacted from other children or pets.

Tinea capitis - hair loss and scale

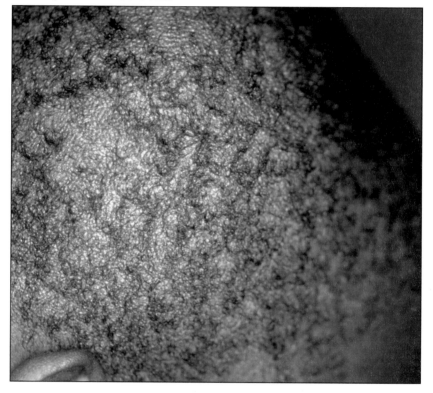

The appearance of the rash and the degree of scale and inflammation in the scalp depends on which fungus is involved. Scale and hair loss is a common feature. Some species produce a black dot appearance from broken hairs. At the other end of the spectrum cattle ringworm can cause a very severe pustular reaction. A kerion is a fungal infection of the scalp that is associated with severe inflammation, progressing to scarring.

If tinea capitis is suspected samples should be taken for mycology, including scale and hair. A Wood's light can be used as a screening test for tinea capitis. However, only some of the species of dermatophytes that cause tinea capitis fluoresce under a Wood's light. A local laboratory may offer a mycology service and some even collect the samples. Specimens include skin scrapings and hairs. Another method is to rub a toothbrush on the scalp to collect a sample for mycology.

> **Tip:** If the diagnosis of a scaly scalp is in doubt send samples for mycology

Diffuse hair loss

Iron deficiency and thyroid disease can cause hair diffuse hair loss. It is therefore worth checking an FBC, ferritin and TFT in cases. Increasing hair shedding can occur some months after a major event such as pregnancy or systemic illness (telogen effluvium). Some drugs can cause hair loss, including ACE inhibitors, anticoagulants and cytotoxics.

Hair loss is most common as male pattern baldness, with frontal recession and hair loss from the crown. There is no scarring and it tends to be familial. Bald men may claim to be more virile, but possibly get less chance to prove it! Female pattern (androgenetic) alopecia is quite common in middle-aged women and there is often a positive family history (takes after mother)! There is thinning of the scalp hair, but preservation of the normal hairline. There is no scarring. It is worth checking a serum testosterone to exclude an endocrine disease.

Localised hair loss without scarring

Alopecia areata presents as localised shiny areas of hair loss. The surface of the scalp is normal, in contrast to scarring alopecia and tinea capitis. There are exclamation hairs at the periphery of the lesions. These are hairs that narrow to their base. As the hair re-grows, fine white hairs appear. There can be total loss of scalp hair (alopecia totalis). Other sites can be affected such as the eyebrows, beard, axillary and pubic area. The nails can be pitted nails. There is an association with autoimmune diseases and it is worth checking autoantibodies, TFT and a RBS. Extensive disease or early onset is associated with a poorer prognosis.

Traction for hair rollers can produce hair loss. Hair plucking (trichotillomania) is usually seen in young females, with areas of hair loss in the margins of the scalp, often with a few hairs remaining.

Alopecia areata - hair loss with normal scalp

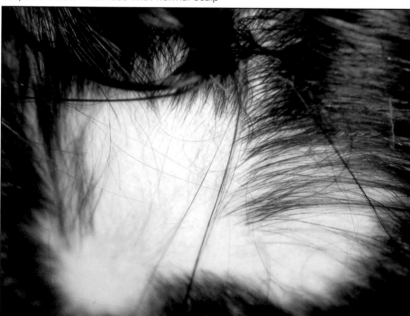

Localised hair loss with scarring

Scarring alopecia is uncommon. It can be due to discoid lupus or lichen planus. The scarring itself can be quite subtle and can easily be misdiagnosed as alopecia areata. The term pseudopelade is applied to scarring alopecia with minimal inflammation. With scarring alopecia the hair does not re-grow. Looking for a rash at other sites can help with diagnosis; however, there is often a need for a punch biopsy to provide histology. Other causes of scarring alopecia include trauma (burns, radiotherapy) and tumours.

Scarring alopecia - hair loss and scalp scarring

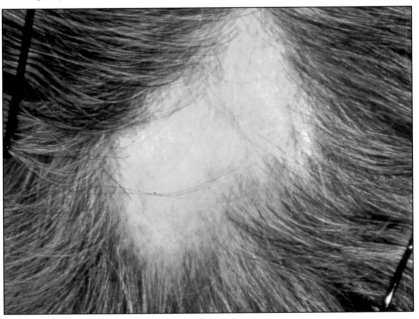

The bald scalp of the elderly male is a very common site of solar damage. There are frequently actinic keratoses and occasionally squamous cell carcinomas. In folliculitis decalvans there is a severe bacterial infection of the scalp with deep-seated pustules and again this goes on and scars.

Excess hair

Excess hair can be localised or generalised. Hirsutism is a male pattern hair growth in the female. In its mildest form females complain of excess hair on the upper lip. It is rarely due to any hormonal problem. Key questions in the history include are the periods normal, is there any family history of this problem, any deepening of the voice or galactorrhoea?

When there is any endocrine problem, then it is usually polycystic ovary syndrome. Other rare possibilities include adrenal and ovarian tumours, pituitary tumours and drugs. Screening tests include U&E, RBS, testosterone, DHEAS, FSH and LH and prolactin. Patients with PCOS have a slightly elevated testosterone, whilst those with tumours have much higher levels.

Tip: With hair problems always ask about family history.

Trunk and limbs

When trying to diagnose rashes on the trunk and limbs, do not get too close too early. Do look at the distribution of the rash. Does it involve just the trunk, or does it also affect the limbs? It if does involve the limbs, is it primarily the flexor surfaces eg atopic eczema, or the extensors eg psoriasis.

Is the rash symmetrical or asymmetrical? Symmetry would suggest more of an endogenous aetiology whilst asymmetry could be due to allergy or infection. Is the rash itchy and how itchy is it eg lichen planus is very itchy. Are there excoriations from scratching? Is more than one member of the family scratching eg scabies? What colour is the rash? Is it scaly, as this would suggest the disease affects the epidermis? Are there any blisters? Do the lesions have a well-defined border?

The unusual presentation of a common disease presents more frequently than a rare disease. If you see an unusual rash, do look to see if it affects other sites and if these areas look similar to a common skin disease.

> **Tip:** Do not use topical steroids until you have a working diagnosis, as this just makes reaching a final diagnosis even more difficult.

Scaly rashes

Dry itchy skin

Dry scaly skin is very common. It can be due to a congenital ichthyosis, when there is scale but no redness. Ichthyosis vulgaris is the most common, is the mildest and tends to spare the flexures. Patients with atopic eczema have a background of dry skin (xeroderma) but without the degree of scale associated with an ichthyosis. They also have an itchy scaly rash in

Atopic eczema - dry skin and scaly rash in front of elbows

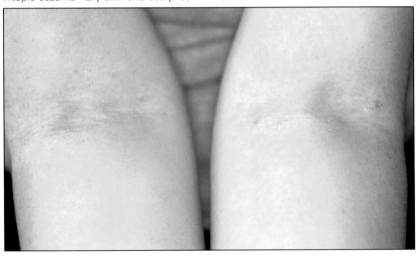

front of the elbows and behind the knees. Patients with both atopic eczema and ichthyosis vulgaris can have small rough papules, especially on their upper arms (keratosis pilaris) and these are more easily felt than seen.

The elderly frequently have dry, itchy skin. This is due to older skin holding fluid less well, the use of abrasive soaps and taking oral diuretics. General medical conditions can also cause itchy, dry skin. Conditions include lymphoma, Hodgkin's disease, polycythaemia, renal disease, hepatic problems and thyroid disease. It is well worth doing some screening investigations before referring. Secondary care can frequently do no more and the GP, after initial investigation, can make the most appropriate referral first time.

Atopic eczema/dermatitis (see also common rashes on page 21)

Atopic eczema presents as an itchy, symmetrical, erythematous rash in the creases at the elbows, knees and ankles. The persistent scratching can produce lichenification. Secondary infection with weeping and pustulation is common.

Eczema - itchy red excoriated scaly rash

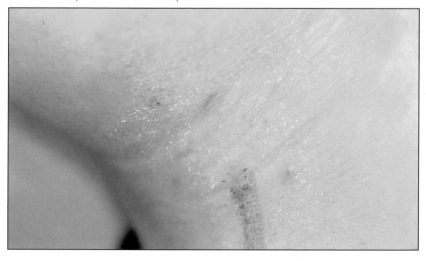

Lichen simplex chronicus

This is the development of scaly lichenified plaques develop at sites of repeated scratching. The skin markings are increased. Favourite sites are the neck, lower leg and genitalia.

> **Tip:** The sites of lichen simplex reflect the areas that can be reached and scratched by the dominant hand.

Itchy skin

Scabies (see common diseases on page 42)

Scabies is a common problem especially in school children and elderly patients in residential homes. The recent development of an itchy rash in a patient or family should alert the GP to the possibility of scabies. There

Itchy rash with burrows in finger webs

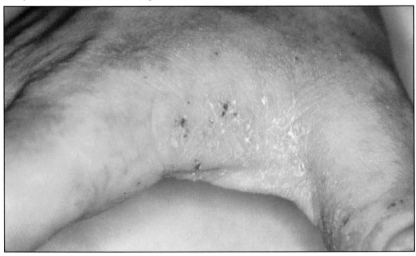

is an itchy, non-specific rash. Common sites are the hands, wrists, axillae and peri-umbilical area, with papules and excoriations. Burrows may be found on the sides and webs of the fingers and wrists. Penile lesions in the male are diagnostic.

Prurigo nodularis

The patient has a very itchy rash, consisting of multiple hyperpigmented nodules. Common sites are the arms, legs and trunk. Scratching is a major factor, with sparing of the area on the back that cannot be reached.

Nodular prurigo - very itchy nodules

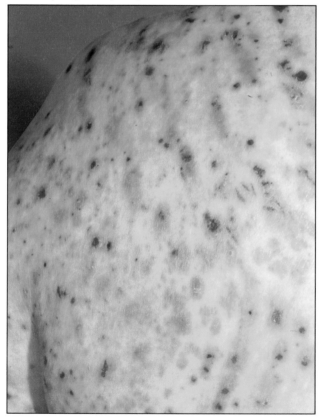

Papulosquamous rashes

These are rashes with scaly lesions that have a well-defined margin.

- Psoriasis, lichen planus, Reiters syndrome

- Pityriasis rubra pilaris, pityriasis rosea, pityriasis lichenoides

- Pityriasis versicolor, tinea

- Drug eruptions (see common skin diseases on page 42)

- Chronic superficial dermatitis

Psoriasis (see common rashes on page 34)

Psoriasis presents with symmetrical scaly plaques on the elbows, knees and lower back. The scale is silvery and the plaques have a well defined edge. There can be scalp and nail involvement. Guttate psoriasis

Scalp psoriasis - scaly red rash without hair loss

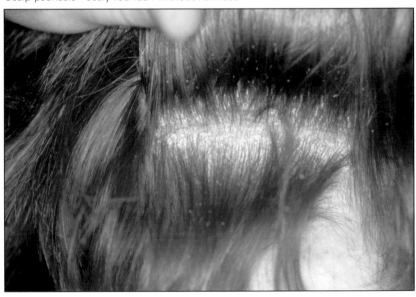

classically presents in childhood or adolescence following a streptococcal sore throat. There is an extensive rash consisting of small, scaly, raindrop-like lesions.

Lichen planus (LP)

This is an inflammatory skin disease. Drug induced lichenoid eruptions are very similar in appearance. The most common site for lichen planus is at the wrists. There are violaceous flat-topped polygonal papules with white streaks on their surface (Wickham's striae). Lichen planus can present as hypertrophic plaques on the shins. When lichen planus resolves it leaves purple staining of the skin, which can be useful to give a late diagnosis.

Lichen planus - flat topped papules with white streaks

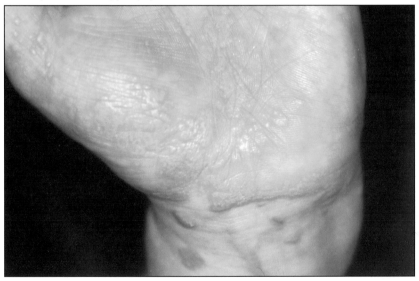

The buccal mucosa can be involved with a fine lace-like pattern. In the scalp there can be scarring alopecia. The nails are frequently involved with loss of the nail plate. Lichen planus on the hands tends to look like psoriasis. Lichen nitidus can be regarded as a variant of lichen planus, but with smaller lesions.

> **Tip:** *If you suspect lichen planus do look in the mouth.*

Pityriasis rosea

This disease is most common in young adults although it can occur at any age. It is more common in the spring and autumn and is probably of viral aetiology, although this is not proven. There is an initial larger erythematous, scaly, herald patch on the trunk. This can be mistaken for tinea corporis. The author has taken scrapings for mycology only to see the general rash appear a few days later. The general rash follows two to

Pityriasis rosea - oval patches with fir tree distribution

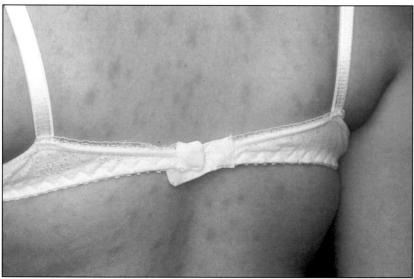

four days after the herald patch. There are oval, petaloid patches following the ribs in a fir tree distribution. The rash can spread down onto the upper arms and thighs, but rarely down onto the hands and feet. If it does so, do think – could this be syphilis!

The lesions of pityriasis rosea have a very characteristic collarette of scale. The rash resolves after approximately six weeks. Pityriasis rosea can present as a papular rash and the differential diagnosis includes guttate psoriasis.

Tip: When faced with a bizarre rash, don't forget that the following: SLE, syphilis, and drug rashes, can masquerade in a multitude of disguises.

Pityriasis lichenoides

This is found in children and young adults. There are acute and chronic forms. The rash can present as pink papules and vesicles, resembling chickenpox that does not resolve. Another presentation is an itchy rash on the trunk and limbs, especially gluteal region, composed of small reddish-brown scaly papules. The scale can be picked off in one.

Pityriasis rubra pilaris (PRP)

This is an uncommon condition that affects the scalp, trunk and palms. The scalp is red and scaly. The rash on the trunk is red, scaly and has islands of sparing. The palms are thickened and yellow.

Reiter's disease

The patient has a psoriasiform rash. Other features include a urethritis, conjunctivitis and arthritis. The penis can have a balanitis with a circinate edge.

Pityriasis versicolor

This is due to the yeast Malassezia furfur. The rash takes the form of fawn or brown patches on the trunk. The rash is slightly scaly, which helps distinguish it from vitiligo. To pale skin they are hyperpigmented, whilst on dark skin they are hypopigmented. This is because the fungus inhibits the skin's normal pigmentation by producing carboxylic acid.

Pityriasis versicolor - scaly patches

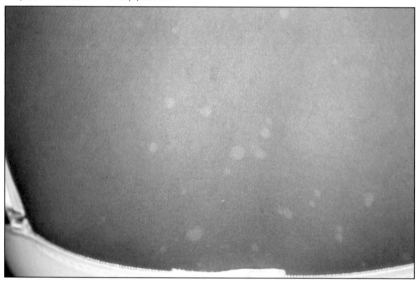

Tinea corporis

Tinea corporis presents as red, annular lesions with an active, scaly border. There is often tinea at other sites eg tinea pedis. Diagnosis is confirmed by taking skin scrapings for mycology.

Chronic superficial dermatitis

This presents as very superficial scaly patches on the trunk and thighs. As the name suggests, they look eczematous. The patches are uniform and can have a finger-like appearance. Most cases run a benign course and it is now thought that this rash very rarely progresses.

Chronic superficial dermatitis - superficial scaly patches

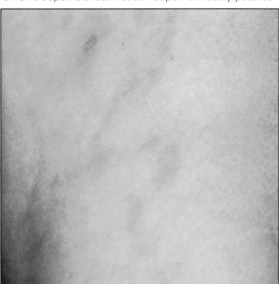

Mycosis fungoides

This is a T-cell lymphoma of the skin. The disease presents in the middle aged or elderly with very itchy, often slightly asymmetrical, well demarcated patches on the trunk. There can be poikiloderma (atrophy telangiectasia and reticulate pigmentation). The disease progresses to plaques, then nodules and ulceration. Eventually there is hepatosplenomegaly and lymphadenopathy.

> ***Tip:*** *The GP should consider whether this could be early mycosis fungoides, when a presumed 'eczema', 'psoriasis', or 'fungal infection' is atypical or refractory to treatment.*

Non-scaly rashes on the trunk and limbs

Urticaria (also see common diseases on page 37)

Urticaria is also known as nettle rash or hives. The patient has a transient itchy rash that is composed of wheals (raised white lesions from oedema). Urticaria beyond six weeks can be regarded as chronic. With urticaria it is worth inquiring about any new medication, any relationship to food or any association with temperature or exercise.

The annular erythemas

This term can be used to include a number of red rashes with an annular border. Scaling is variable.

Granuloma annulare

Common sites are the backs of the hands and dorsum of the feet. This presents as a red patch with a raised border. The lack of scale helps

Granuloma annulare - raised border without scale

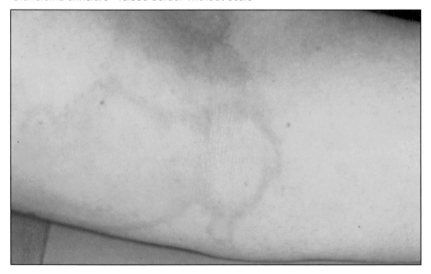

distinguish the rash from tinea. Only the diffuse form is associated with diabetes mellitus.

Erythema multiforme

Erythema multiforme can be triggered by herpes simplex and drugs. The classical 'target iris-like' lesions are red in colour and exhibit central clearing. Stephens Johnson syndrome is a more severe form of erythema multiforme with mucosal involvement.

Erythema multiforme - can be bullous and haemorrhagic

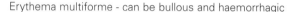

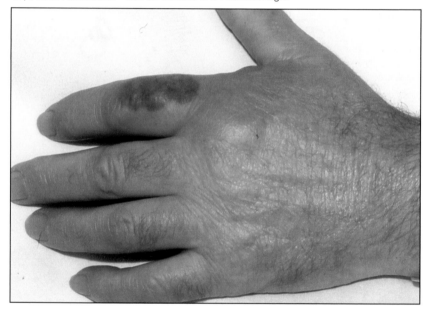

Deposits in the skin

Uric acid

In gout, apart from the joint problems, uric acid can be deposited in the ears and fingers. These present as hard yellow subcutaneous nodules.

Calcium

Calcium is deposited in the fingers in some of the collagen diseases eg the CREST syndrome (calcinosis cutis). There are hard white papules in the extremities. Children sometimes develop a solitary hard papule on the face (cutaneous calculus).

Cholesterol

A raised cholesterol and lipids is common in primary care. However, many of the skin manifestations are uncommon. Xanthelasma are found around the eyes as yellow plaques. Eruptive xanthoma present as yellow papules and nodules on the trunk. Xanthoma can also present over bony prominences such as the elbows. The palms and soles can have lipid deposits. The tendency to xanthoma can be inherited or secondary to systemic disease. It is important to screen the patient for thyroid, liver, renal or pancreatic disease.

Eruptive xanthoma - red/yellow deposits of lipid

Tests include:

- cholesterol, HDL and fasting lipids

- U&E, RBS, TFT, LFTs

- Urine dipstick

Changes in pigmentation (vitiligo, morphoea, lichen sclerosus et atrophicus)

A change in skin pigmentation is a frequent consultation. Injury to the skin can result in hyperpigmentation or hypopigmentation. Eczema and acne are common diseases that can produce pigmentary changes. The primary rash gives the diagnosis. Pityriasis versicolor results in fawn coloured slightly scaly patches. Lichen planus goes on to leave mauve staining.

Vitiligo presents as white patches with a normal skin texture and surface. In morphoea there are localised thickened pale patches. As the name

Vitiligo - areas of depigmentaton

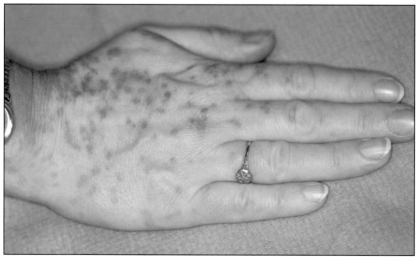

would suggest the white patches of lichen sclerosus et atrophicus are atrophic. An orange discoloration of the skin occurs in carotenaemia, due to eating too many carrots or drinking excessive amounts of orange juice.

Rashes with blistering

Blistering can cause alarm bells to ring, and GPs often immediately think of the inflammatory bullous diseases. However, many common rashes can blister. Blistering can be a feature of: trauma, insect bites, infection, acute eczema, drug rashes (eg sulphonamides and barbiturates) and erythema multiforme. Blisters can occur on oedematous legs and these are not associated with inflammation.

Blister - insect bite

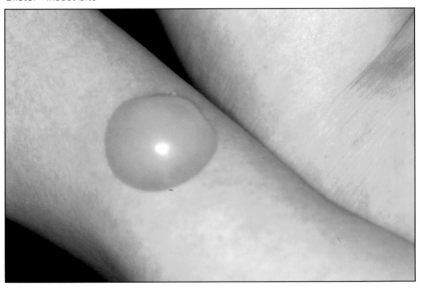

Blistering due to infection

Impetigo can blister then form a yellow crust. Herpes simplex lesions around the mouth present with initial pain, then vesiculation. Shingles is due to reactivation of the varicella-zoster virus. After some initial pain a rash develops along a dermatome. The rash consists of blisters on an erythematous base. Secondary infection can lead to the rash becoming impetiginized. Tinea pedis can also blister.

Blisters and eczema/dermatitis

Blistering can be a feature of an acute eczema. Pompholyx, a type of eczema has vesicles and blisters. A phytophotodermatitis occurs when sap from the giant hogweed plant is splashed onto a limb that is exposed to sunlight. There is a rash composed of linear vesicular streaks.

Epidermolysis bullosa (EB)

These are a group of inherited blistering disorders in response to minimal trauma. They vary in severity and some can be fatal.

Epidermolysis bullosa - inherited blistering disorder

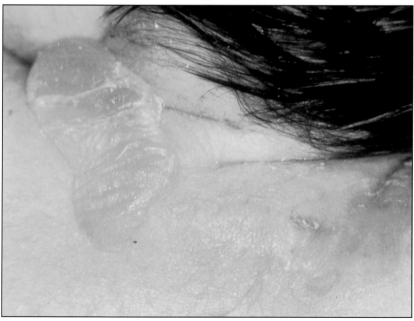

Dermatitis herpetiformis

Dermatitis herpetiformis presents with very itchy, small blisters on the shoulders, elbows, knees and gluteal region. It is associated with gluten enteropathy and endomysial antibodies.

Pemphigus

Pemphigus vulgaris usually affects the 40 to 60 age group. There is blistering of the skin and mucous membranes. The blisters are very superficial and are soon lost leaving eroded areas. When unaffected skin is rubbed it blisters; this is known as Nikolsky's sign. Pemphigus vulgaris can cause painful oral ulceration. Pemphigus foliaceus presents as weeping, crusted areas on the head and neck.

Pemphigoid

Bullous pemphigoid affects the over-60 age group. There can be an initial urticated rash before the blisters appear. Bullous pemphigoid affects the trunk and spares the face, hands and mucous membranes. Cicatricial pemphigoid (benign mucous membrane pemphigoid) involves the eyes, mouth and genitalia. It results in severe scarring that is certainly not benign!

Linear IgA disease

This can resemble bullous pemphigoid. However, there is an abrupt onset of annular lesions and there is mucosal involvement. Chronic bullous dermatosis of childhood resembles linear IgA disease in adults. Blisters are found on the genitalia, gluteal region and inner thighs. The term linear IgA refers to the band of immunofluorescence seen on biopsy.

Porphyria cutanea tarda

Porphyria presents with sun-induced blisters on exposed sites. On the backs of the hands there are blisters and scars. The urine fluoresces pink under a Wood's light. Blood, urine and stools can be sent for porphyrins. Liver function tests should be performed.

Porphyria - blisters and scars

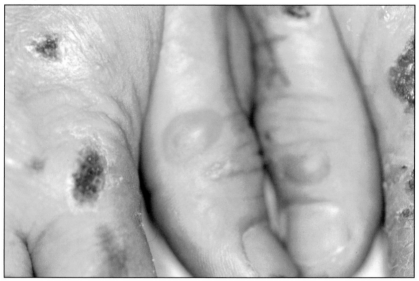

Investigation of bullous disease

With a blistering disease there is the need to send tissue for both histology and direct immunofluorescence. Indirect immunofluorescence on serum is possible, but less reliable. Blood can also be sent for endomysial antibodies in dermatitis herpetiformis, an immunology screen including an ANA for lupus, and blood, urine and faeces for porphyrins.

Rashes that seem to turn up in meetings and examinations!

There are certain rashes that, whilst rare at a primary care consultation, appear frequently in meetings and examinations. Not infrequently the patient has had the rash for many years and has never bothered to inquire about it. At some time they may have been given the correct or incorrect diagnosis.

Erythemas

Erythema chronicum migrans (Lyme disease)

This is due to infection with the spirochaete Borrelia burgdorferi, following a bite from a tick. An annular, red patch with central clearing develops around the site of the bite. Later sequelae include arthritis, cardiac and neurological complications.

Erythema annulare centrifugum

- Can be associated with malignancy and drugs
- Red annular lesions
- Can have a scaly border

Erythema gyratum repens

- Associated with malignant disease
- Pronounced annular erythema
- Wave-like pattern
- Resembles wood grain
- Rapid progression

Erythema elevatum diutinum

- Wrists, elbows and knees
- Pink or purple plaques/nodules
- Rash can scar

Erythema marginatum

- ■ Associated with rheumatic fever

- ■ Usually on trunk

- ■ Annular erythema

- ■ Transient and easily missed

Connective tissue diseases

Livedo reticularis - note net-like pattern

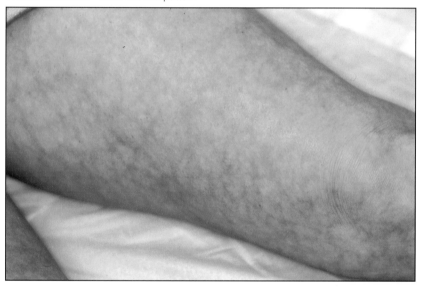

Scleroderma

This can be localised as morphoea or generalised as systemic sclerosis. Morphoea presents as thickened shiny patches of skin with hair loss. In systemic sclerosis patients develop taut, shiny skin over the hands (sclerodactyly). They can have systemic involvement.

CREST syndrome

- Calcinosis

- Raynaud's phenomenon

- Oesophageal dysmotility

- Scleroderma

- Telangiectasia

Lichen sclerosus et atrophicus

- Usually females

- White, atrophic patches

- Telangiectasia

- Can affect the vulva

Dermatomyositis

- 20 per cent have a malignancy

- Rash and myopathy

- Mauve (heliotrope) rash around the eyes

- Backs of the hands violaceous papules (Gottron's papules)

- Nail fold changes of telangiectasia & infarcts

Granulomatous diseases

Sarcoid

- Granulomatous disease

- Papular or nodular

- Can occur in scars

- Can have systemic involvement

Sarcoid - extensive erythematous rash without scale

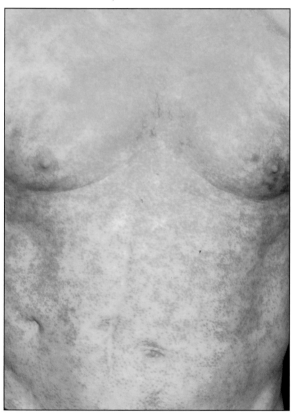

Inherited diseases

Xeroderma pigmentosum

- Autosomal recessive

- Defective DNA repair

- Photosensitivity

- Skin cancers

- Can be fatal

Neurofibromatosis

- Autosomal dominant with variable penetrance

- Café au lait spots

- Axilliary freckling

- Multiple neurofibroma – soft nodules, feel 'button holed' into the skin

Tuberous sclerosis

- Autosomal dominant

- Adenoma sebaceum – pink papules on nose and cheeks

- Ash-leaf macules – oval hypopigmented patches

- Shagreen patches – naevi over lumbosacral area

- Peri-ungual fibromas

Darier's disease

- Autosomal dominant
- Rash exacerbated by sunshine
- Neck, chest and back
- Brown, scaly papules
- Palms and soles have pits and punctate keratoses
- Nails have longitudinal ridges

Ehlers-Danlos syndrome

- Increased tissue fragility and extensibility
- Prominent in the neck
- 'Cigarette paper' scars over bony prominences.
- Scars resulting from minor trauma
- Joint hyper extensibility

Pseudoxanthoma elasticum

- Autosomal recessive or dominant
- Yellow wrinkled skin
- Small papules
- 'Chicken skin' appearance

Malignancy

Sezary syndrome

- Elderly males.

- Itchy erythroderma

- Sezary cells (large convoluted nucleus)

- Sezary cells in the skin and blood.

Great mimic

Secondary syphilis

- Copper coloured scaly rash

- Lymphadenopathy, alopecia

- Mouth – snail track ulcers

- Anogenital area – condylomata lata

Flexures and concealed areas

Flexures

Some rashes occur only in the flexures, whilst others are also found at other sites but are modified by being in the flexures. The flexures are sites where two folds of skin come into contact. The friction between the two surfaces reduces the amount of scale. The heat and maceration predisposes to secondary infection.

Flexural psoriasis - red rash with well defined border

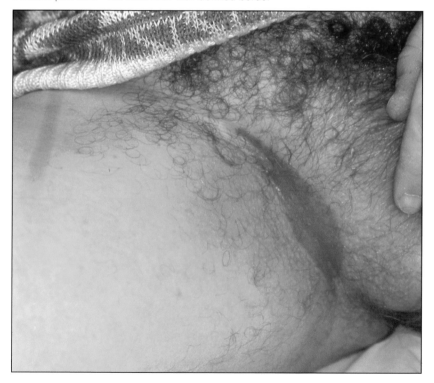

Intertrigo

Intertrigo is produced in the flexures by the warm moist environment. The red moist rash frequently is secondarily infected. Candida infection is common and this can be diagnosed by the presence of satellite pustules. It is worth taking swabs for bacteria and candida.

Intertrigo - flexural rash with secondary infection

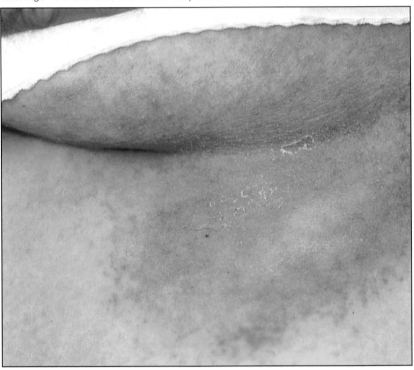

Nappy rash

This is an irritant dermatitis. Satellite papules indicate secondary infection with candida. Erosive changes suggest prolonged contact with soiled nappies.

Psoriasis and seborrhoeic dermatitis

Psoriasis in the flexures is still red and has a well-defined border, but there is far less scale than on the trunk. The uniformity of the rash and the absence of a raised edge help distinguish this rash from tinea cruris. Seborrhoeic dermatitis localises to the flexures with an eczematous rash that is frequently secondarily infected.

Tinea cruris

Tinea cruris is found in the groins, usually in male patients. They invariably also have tinea pedis. There is a rash with a raised scaly edge and central clearing.

Tinea cruris - rash in groins with raised scaly border

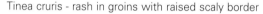

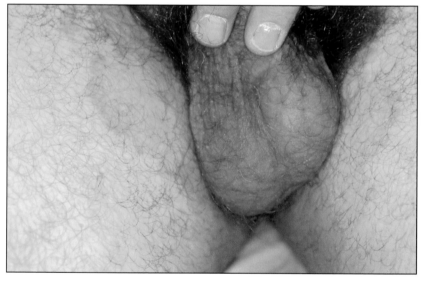

> **Tip:** The presence of scale helps differentiate tinea at any site from granuloma annulare.

Erythrasma

Erythrasma presents as light brown scaly patches in the axillae and groins. It does not have the raised edge of tinea. Under a Wood's light these areas have a coral red florescence.

Hidradenitis suppurativa

This presents as an acneform rash in the flexures. There is an erythematous rash with painful nodules, abscesses, sinuses and scars.

Hidradenitis suppurativa - nodules, abscess and sinuses

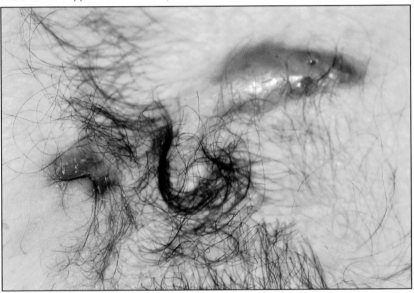

Acanthosis nigricans

There are velvet-like, thickened pigmented areas in the flexures associated with internal malignancy. The surface tends to be rough with numerous tags. Pseudo acanthosis nigricans is associated with obesity and diabetes.

Hyperhidrosis (excessive sweating)

Hyperhidrosis can be generalised or localised to areas such as the axillae, palms and soles. Sweating is a common source of embarrassment. These sites when affected are prone to secondary infection (fungal infections and pitted keratolysis on the feet).

Pitted keratolysis - malodorous feet with pits

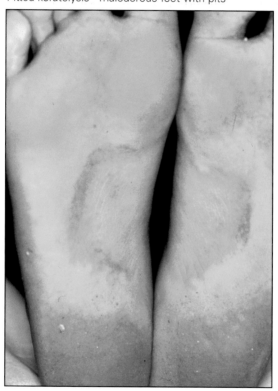

Rashes on the genitalia and perineum

Genital rashes can cause concern and, for some, considerable distress. Many patients try all sorts of OTC medication before they consult. These OTC medications can in turn lead to a contact allergic dermatitis. Some patients do attend 'GU' clinics, although these are not the best place for those whose disease is not sexually transmitted. Many patients with genital rashes abstain from sex as a result of pain, discomfort or embarrassment.

Over recent years many doctors have developed a special interest in genital rashes. When the diagnosis is not obvious do consider referral to the nearest vulval clinic, or to an expert with an interest in male genital rashes.

Candida (thrush) is common and genital warts are not uncommon. Thrush should respond to simple treatment with antifungals and does not scar. Common itchy rashes in the vulva are lichen simplex, seborrhoeic dermatitis, allergic contact eczema and psoriasis.

Seborrhoeic dermatitis - Koebner phenomenon in a scar

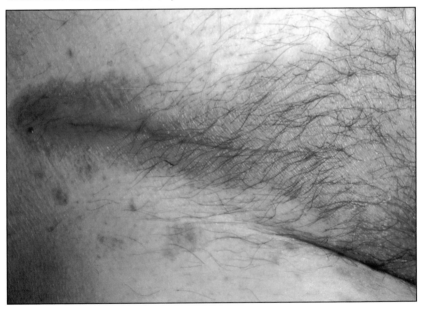

The white vulva can be due to lichen sclerosus and lichen planus. Lichen sclerosus presents as white itchy patches with atrophy. It can predispose to malignancy. Lichen planus is very itchy and can have a purple colour.

A rash at other sites can help with the diagnosis, although biopsy is often required.

Lichen simplex - increased skin markings

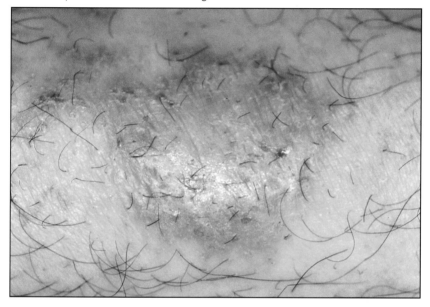

Intraepidermal carcinoma can affect the penis, vulva and peri-anal area. This can present as well defined red patches, plaques or papules. Untreated they can progress to squamous cell carcinoma. Biopsy is needed to confirm or refute the diagnosis.

Consultations for syndromes with a plethora of symptoms and a paucity of signs are not uncommon in these areas eg vulvar vestibulitis, vulvodynia, and burning scrotum syndrome.

Penile rashes are a cause for concern. Pearly penile papules are physiological but misdiagnosed as penile warts. On the corona of the penis are rows of very small papules. Genital warts present as flesh coloured papules. The differential diagnosis includes condylomata lata (syphilis). Other penile rashes are listed below.

Balanitis xerotica obliterans

- Linked to LSA

- White colour

- Superficial atrophy

- Telangiectasia and scarring

Behçet's syndrome

- Oral and genital ulceration

- Erythema nodosum

- Pustules at sites of injury

Bowenoid papulosis

- Intra epithelial neoplasia

- Reddish brown papules

Erythroplasia of Queyrat

- Intra epidermal carcinoma

- Velvet red plaque

- Biopsy for diagnosis

Zoon's balanitis

- Plasma cell balanitis

- Elderly male

- Shiny red plaque

- Biopsy for diagnosis

Pruritus ani

Pruritus ani is a common consultation in general practice and one that frequently fails to reach a diagnosis. When taking the history, do ask about threadworms (a piece of double-sided sticky tape can be left near the anus overnight, to catch and display emerging threadworms). Enquire into the use of OTC topical therapies as they can cause a dermatitis. It is important to examine the patient for an anal fissure or piles. It is also worth looking at other sites for evidence of inflammatory skin conditions such as eczema or psoriasis.

The lower legs

Asteatotic eczema

This presents as a dry, itchy rash on the legs. The rash has crazy-paving appearance. It is associated with a dry environment, myxoedema and diuretics.

Asteatotic eczema - crazy paving appearance

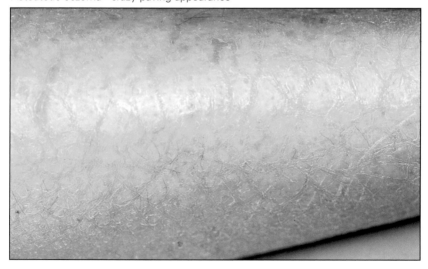

Ulcers

Ulcers are not uncommon on the lower leg. Varicose ulcers are associated with venous insufficiency, oedema, ulceration, pigmentation and an eczematous rash. There can be scarring, white scars (atrophie blanche) and fibrosis (lipodermatosclerosis). Venous ulcers have granulation tissue that bleeds easily and can go on and scar.

Arterial ulcers are smaller, deeper and have a punched-out appearance. The leg is cold, shiny and the skin is rather atrophic. There may be a history of claudication. Tobacco consumption should be recorded. Diabetic neuropathic ulceration occurs at sites of pressure. Using a Doppler to measure the blood pressure in lower and upper limb helps diagnose suspected vascular insufficiency and pick up those with occult disease.

Cellulitis

The commonest pathogen is a haemolytic streptococcus, although *Staph. aureus* is a possibility. A cellulitis presents as a swollen warm tender leg.

Cellulitis - tender warm swollen leg

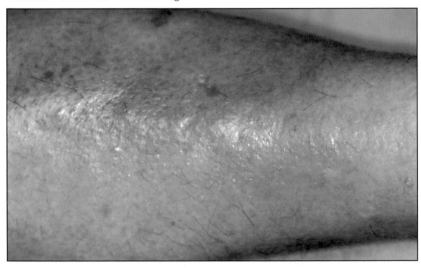

The portal of entry can be from a wound, leg ulcer, or tinea pedis. The differential diagnosis includes a deep vein thrombosis. Tests that help distinguish between a DVT and cellulitis include D-dimers, ultrasonography and a venogram.

Cellulitis - cellulitis with blistering, secondary to tinea pedis

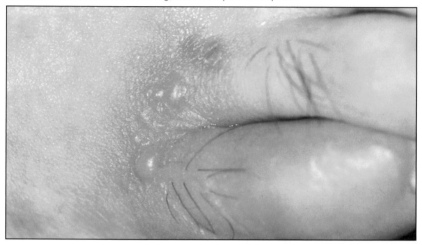

Ecthyma - localised infection

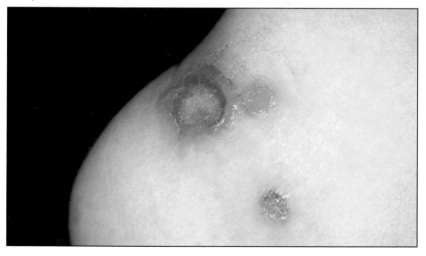

Pyoderma gangrenosum

This presents as a tender red nodule that breaks down to form an ulcer with an overhanging purplish edge. The ulcer has a necrotic base. It is associated with inflammatory bowel disease.

Purpura

Erythematous purpuric rash -
lower leg

Purpura -
black non blanching rash

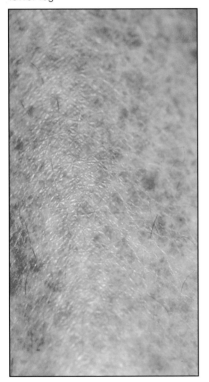 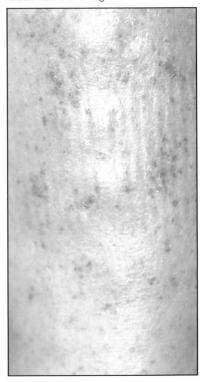

The lower legs are a favourite site for purpura. This may be due to a problem with platelets or vessels. A vasculitis presents as painful palpable purpura whilst a capillaritis as fine non-palpable purpura.

Henoch Schoenlein purpura

This is a small vessel vasculitis that can be precipitated by a Streptococcal sore throat. It presents with painful, palpable purpura on the buttocks and legs.

Erythema nodosum

This is a panniculitis. It presents as painful, tender, red nodules on the lower shins. Some cases are associated with streptococcal infections. Other causes include the granulomatous disease (sarcoidosis and TB), inflammatory bowel disease (Crohn's disease and ulcerative colitis), and drugs (oral contraceptives and sulphonamides).

Erythema nodosum - tender red nodules

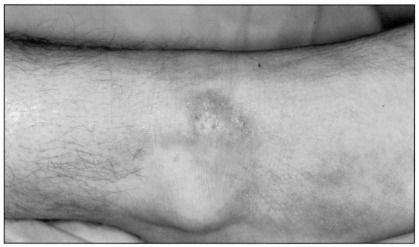

Erythema ab igne

- Can be due to heat

- Lower legs

- Net-like pigmented erythema

Pigmented purpuric eruption

- Capillaritis – tiny petechiae
- Lower legs
- Itchy, orange-brown rash

Erythema induratum

- Associated with chronic infection eg TB
- Backs of the lower legs
- Purple, ulcerating nodules

Necrobiosis lipoidica

- Associated with diabetes
- Lower legs
- Shiny patches
- Yellow centre and a red edge

Necrobiosis lipoidica - shiny yellow patches on lower legs

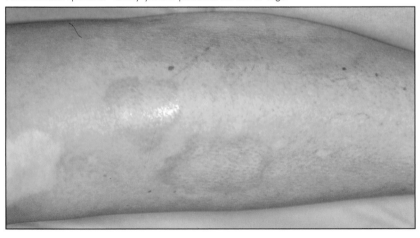

Bowen's disease

- Intra-epidermal squamous cell carcinoma

- Red, scaly patch

Angiokeratoma

- Haemangioma

- Scaly surface

Stucco keratoses

- Variant of seborrhoeic keratoses

- Lower legs

- White, hyperkeratotic papules

Hands and Feet

The hands

The hands are a part of the body that frequently come into contact with the outside world. They, like the face are an area exposed to sunshine. Some rashes tend to affect only the hands, whilst others the feet, but many affect both. When trying to diagnose rashes on the hands taking a good history is essential. Key points are – are there rashes at other sites, which is the dominant hand, what tasks are performed with each hand, what is the occupation and hobbies. Do include examination of the nails with examination of the hands.

Eczematous rashes on the hands and feet

Irritant contact dermatitis is more common than allergic contact dermatitis. Atopics are more prone to an irritant dermatitis as are workers in certain occupations. This may be because of contact with greases, solvents, or the hands constantly being in water.

Classic sites for an irritant dermatitis are the web spaces of the fingers. The pulps of the fingers can be affected in both irritant and allergic dermatitis from foods. However, no pattern totally distinguishes irritant from allergic contact dermatitis.

Pointers towards allergic contact dermatitis are a well-defined edge to the rash due to a glove, or asymmetry of the rash. Allergic contact dermatitis to footwear can give a rash with a well-defined edge. Patch testing is frequently required to help exclude an allergic component.

Hyperkeratotic eczema presents as a red, itchy rash on the hands and feet. The rash is scaly and lichenified. The lack of silvery scale and the

Tinea on the palms - unilateral scaly rash

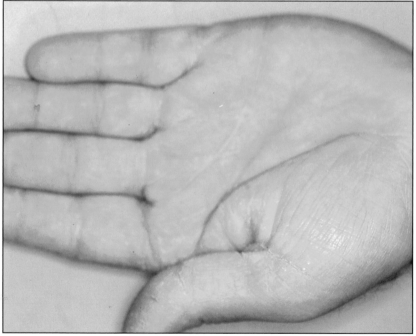

absence of lesions at other sites help distinguish this from psoriasis. Tinea on the palms (Tinea manuum) presents as a dry, scaly palm.

Thickened skin on the hands and feet

Thickened palms and soles occur in many conditions including eczema, lichen planus, psoriasis, pityriasis rubra pilaris, Reiter's disease, and keratoderma. Patients with Reiter's disease can also have a psoriasiform rash on the palms and soles. Keratoderma presents with thickened skin with fissures. It can be inherited, or related to systemic disease, such as carcinoma of oesophagus.

Warts and verrucae are very common, especially in children. Warts present as rough uniform papules and nodules in the hands, whilst verrucae present as flat, tender lesions on the soles of the feet, with thrombosed capillaries within them. Thickening over the knuckles (knuckle pads) does tend to run in families and may be related to repeated trauma. Callosities (corns) are common over sites of pressure. Actinic keratoses are often found on the backs of hands of Caucasians that have had a lot of sun exposure.

Blistering rashes on the hands and feet

A solitary, painful, vesicular lesion on a finger would point to herpes simplex. Such lesions are not uncommon on the fingers of people in certain occupations eg dentists. Any acute hand eczema can contain vesicles and blisters. Pompholyx is a type of eczema that affects the hands and feet. It presents as a red, itchy rash with vesicles and bullae. The rash starts with vesicles on the palms and sides of the fingers that enlarge to become bullae. Allergic contact dermatitis can produce a similar picture.

Localised pustular psoriasis of the hands and feet

This is usually found in middle aged female smokers. There is a red rash on the hands and feet. There are sterile pustules that are either yellow or brown. Tinea pedis can blister and taking samples for mycology helps reach the right diagnosis.

Localised pustular psoriasis - sterile yellow/brown pustules

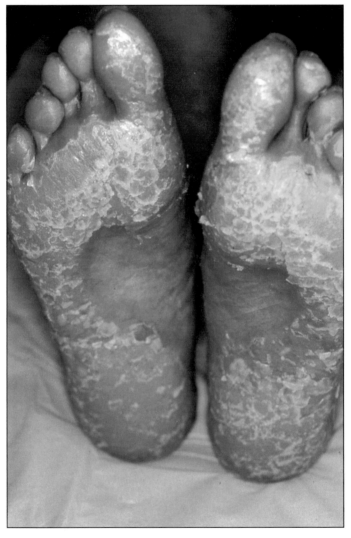

Itchy scaly feet

Tinea, eczema and psoriasis can produce itchy, red feet. Tinea usually presents as an itchy erythematous rash that starts in the space between the 4th and 5th toes. It can also produce vesicles and pustules in the instep. There is a more extensive form known as moccasin type. Tinea on the feet can produce a secondary rash on the palms. Small blisters on the palms appear as part of an immunological reaction, this being known as an id reaction. Juvenile plantar dermatosis presents as shiny, itchy feet. Pitted keratolysis presents in young people with malodorous, sweaty feet with pits.

Juvenile plantar dermatosis - shiny soles

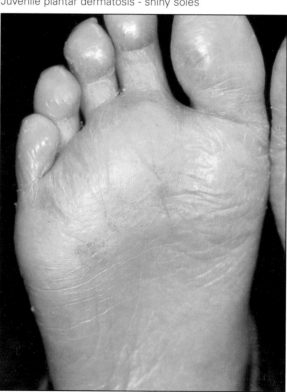

Raynaud's disease (phenomenon)

Raynaud's is when the extremities, that is usually the fingers and toes, go white, then blue to red. There is pain, numbness and tingling. A sudden decrease in temperature can provoke attacks. Many cases are idiopathic but some are secondary to scleroderma, systemic lupus and rheumatoid disease. Use of vibration tools and presence of a cervical rib can produce a similar clinical picture.

Nails

Many GPs have difficulty diagnosing nail disease. Most nail deformities seen in primary care are due to:

- psoriasis, lichen planus

- infection
  (bacterial and fungal)

- trauma

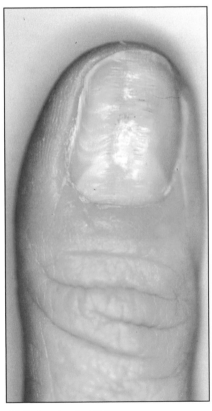

One should look to see if the nail deformity primarily affects the proximal or distal nail. Then one should look at the actual state of the nails. Are they thickened eg psoriasis or tinea. Are there any pits eg psoriasis, lichen planus and alopecia area. Is there any separation of the distal nail from the bed; this is known as onycholysis. Onycholysis is

Nail showing habit tic

found in psoriasis, tinea and tetracycline-induced nail disease.

Other less common signs are black discoloration or pigmentation. This can be due to trauma, a melanoma or racial variation. A green discoloration of the nails occurs in pseudomonas aeruginosa infection. Any systemic illness can affect nail growth, producing Beau's lines. Abnormal nail fold capillaries occur in the connective tissue diseases.

When trying to diagnose nail disease do take nail clippings for mycology. Do take a swab for bacteria and yeasts. When the nail gives the impression of being pushed upwards consider requesting an x-ray to exclude a subungual exostosis.

Psoriasis

Psoriasis presents with thickened nails. There is pitting and onycholysis. There are pink areas known as salmon patches.

Psoriatic nails - thickened, onycholysis and pits

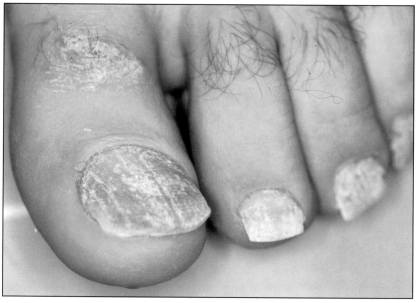

Onychomycosis

This usually presents as a distal nail dystrophy. The nails are thickened with onycholysis and hyperkeratosis. Tinea can also present as a superficial white onychomycosis.

Onychomycosis - yellow nails with onycholysis

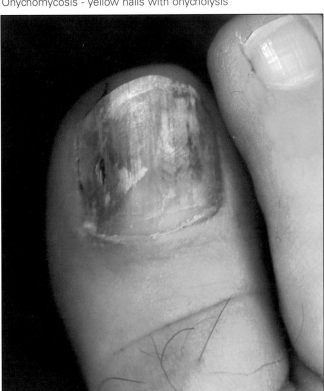

Acute paronychia

There is erythema and swelling of the nail fold, progressing to pus formation. Do take a swab, as there is bacterial infection; this is usually due to *Staph. aureus.*

Chronic paronychia

This is common on those who frequently have their hands in water. There is a swollen nail fold with loss of the cuticle seal. The adjacent nail is ridged and discoloured. Candida is a common pathogen.

Onychomycosis and paronychia

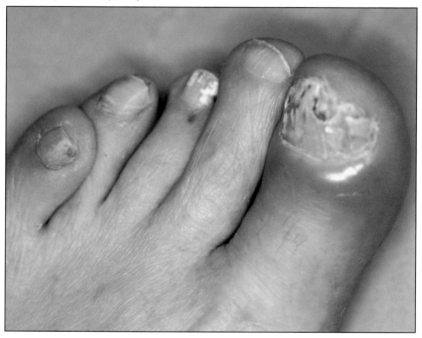

Trauma

Trauma to nails results in subungual haematomas. However, often the patient cannot remember the actual trauma. It is vital to distinguish a haematoma from a melanoma. With a subungual haematoma the pigment does not extend beyond the base of the nail fold and does grow out over time. A habit tic presents with a nail with transverse ridges and furrows.

Malignant melanoma

The spread of pigmentation under the proximal nail fold with a melanoma is known as Hutchinson's sign. Any vertical streak in a Caucasian patient should be a cause of concern. An amelanotic melanoma can mimic a pyogenic granuloma, or chronic paronychia.

Swellings around the proximal nail fold

A myxoid cyst presents as a smooth domed swelling in the vicinity of the proximal nail fold and distal interphalangeal joint. It contains jelly like material. A glomus tumour presents as a very tender red-blue lesion beneath the nail plate.

Peri ungual warts

- Rough papules

- Longitudinal nail groves

Peri ungual warts

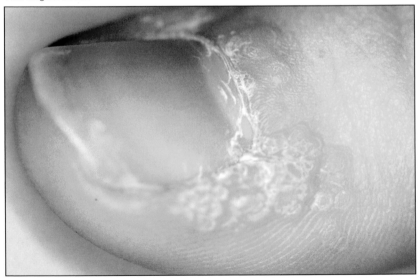

Peri ungual fibroma

■ Arise from nail fold

■ Tuberous sclerosis

Lichen planus

■ Obliteration of the nail fold (pterygium).

■ Longitudinal ridging

■ Pitting.

Yellow nail syndrome

■ Yellow-green nails

■ Over curved nails

■ Association oedema and effusions

Yellow nail syndrome

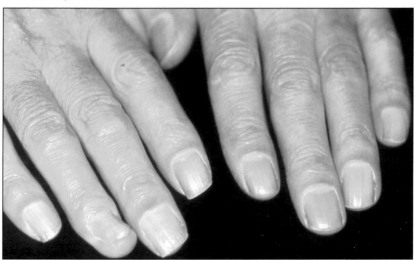

Darier's disease

- Longitudinal ridges
- Notches in the free edge

Part 4

Situations,

occupations

and

special areas

The only lead the GP has might be an occupation, holiday, hobby or sport. This part includes problems related to holidays, hobbies, occupations, pregnancy, psyche, diabetes, transplantation and HIV. Dermatological emergencies are included as, whilst rare, they can put you on the spot.

Holidays, hobbies and sports

Holidays and sport may bring the patient's skin into contact with solar radiation. Since Caucasian skin was probably designed more for the climatic conditions of Manchester or Glasgow, damage easily results. Whilst holidays to the young may be for sun, sand and sin, for the mature age group there is gardening and golf! Any visit to a flower show will reveal the result of the great outdoors, with gardeners covered in actinic keratoses on the backs of their hands and bald heads.

Polymorphic light eruption

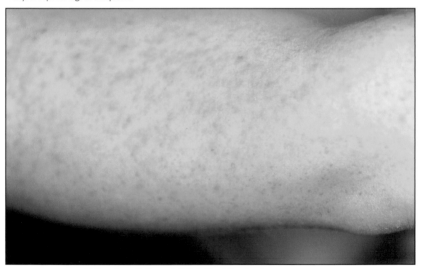

Solar radiation has a major effect on skin diseases. There are a range of solar induced rashes that produce itchy, red rashes on sun exposed sites.

They are, in chronological order, actinic prurigo, juvenile spring eruption, polymorphic light eruption and actinic reticuloid. Teenagers on doxycycline and more mature members of society on thiazides can develop phototoxic reactions. Excessive heat can result in obstructed sweat ducts, prickly heat (miliaria).

Some rashes are aggravated by sunlight such as SLE, DLE, Darier's disease and porphyria. However, many rashes are usually improved by sunlight, such as psoriasis. Whilst patients enjoy sunny days they need to take reasonable precautions and care for their skin!

Insect bites are common in warm climates, with patients consulting because of infected blisters. Larva migrans is due to a hookworm infection. The patient becomes infected after walking barefoot on a tropical beach. There is a slowly expanding tract on the foot.

Insect bite

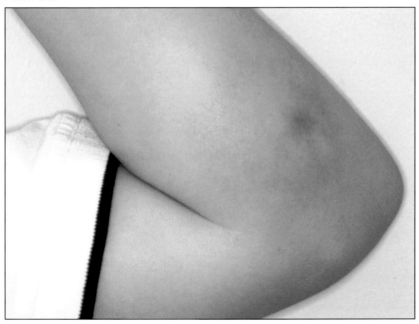

'Spa pool folliculitis' is due to pseudomonas. A few days after bathing in a spa, bath, or Jacuzzi the patient develops tiny itchy papules at sites that were covered by the bathing costume. Sea bather's eruption also affects the bathing suit areas. It is due to stings from the larval form of certain sea anemones and occurs in warm waters. An allergic rash develops a few hours after bathing. 'Swimmers itch' is due to an allergic reaction to immature larval forms of parasitic flatworms. Again, those who travel on exotic holidays are at risk. One to two days after bathing the patient develops an itchy, papular or bullous rash.

Spa pool folliculitis due to pseudomonas

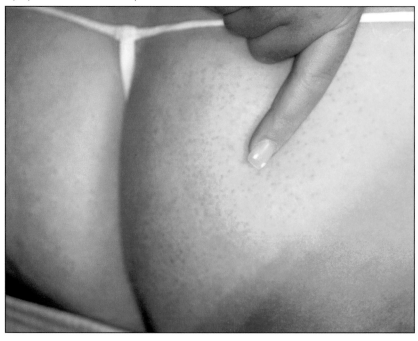

Sport produces heat, sweat, bodily contact and communal bathing. This is just the right environment for the spread of superficial skin infections such as impetigo, tinea cruris, tinea pedis and herpes simplex. Jogging can damage toes with a subungual haematoma under the great toe. Pets are often blamed for allergies and infections. Whilst it is true animal dander can aggravate atopic eczema, a dog may bring a little sanity into a household!

Gardeners are at risk of rashes from plants. A minor irritant dermatitis can develop from contact with plants, soil, water and chemicals. Primula can give a contact allergic dermatitis. A phototoxic reaction occurs when the sap from giant hogweed or rue comes into contact with skin that is then exposed to sunlight. There is acute red rash with blistering.

Fish tank granuloma present in the keepers of tropical fish. This is due to Mycobacterium marinum infection. The patient presents with nodules on the backs of the hands. There is a rash spreading up the lymphatics of the arm (sporotrichoid spread).

Occupational dermatology

An occupational problem is suggested by a rash that is aggravated when working and improves during holidays. Another clue is a rash that develops on taking up a new occupation or multiple employees developing a similar rash. The hands often receive these insults first.

Those with a past history of atopic eczema have a skin less tolerant of insults and more prone to an irritant eczema. The longer the individual works in a particular industry the more likely they are to have a problem. Whilst the use of cleansing agents can be helpful, they should not degrease the skin.

Irritant contact dermatitis is the most common occupational skin problem. Irritant contact eczema frequently affects those in the chemical, petrochemical and construction industries. In the service sector bar staff, catering, cleaning, cooks, domestics, hairdressers and nurses are at risk. Weak irritants include water, soap, saline, weak acids and alkalis, detergents and soluble oils. Strong irritants are bleaches, caustics, paraffin and petroleum.

Allergic contact dermatitis is less common than irritant contact dermatitis. Occupations at increased risk of contact allergic eczema include hairdressers, builders and construction workers. Allergic contact dermatitis to chromate is not uncommon.

People who do a lot of wet work can develop green nails due to pseudomonas nail infections, a chronic paronychia and lamellar splitting (this is when there is flaking of the distal nail).

Those with acne can have their rash exacerbated by oils, greases or hot humid conditions. Butchers are prone to warts on their fingers, whilst dentists can develop herpetic lesions and farmers are at risk of orf.

Rashes in pregnancy

In pregnancy there is a general increase in pigmentation. There can be local increase in pigmentation on the face, known as chloasma. This fades after delivery but can return with oral contraceptives. There is reduced hair loss during pregnancy and then a moult after delivery. Acne can be worse during pregnancy, due to increased sebum production. Increased eccrine glands can cause miliaria. Eczema can improve but may also deteriorate.

Spider naevi are often found on the face and palmar erythema is common. With the increase in abdominal size striae gravidarum and varicose veins are common. Naevi can enlarge and darken, which may cause diagnostic difficulty from melanoma. Non specific itch is quite common in pregnancy. It can be a result of anaemia or intrahepatic cholestasis of pregnancy. Therefore, it is worth checking a FBC, LFTs and bile salts.

Pregnancy and viral infections
(see also 'The Five Ages of Dermatology' - Exanthema in Infancy)

A common consultation is a pregnant female who has come into contact with a child with a viral rash. A rising IgM titre to a specific virus indicates recent infection, whilst a raised IgG implies immunity. Sources of further advice include Microbiologists, Obstetricians, Public health Specialists and Dermatologists.

Most adults are immune to rubella following vaccination, but those females who are not immune are at risk. With regard to chickenpox, many have had the disease in childhood. However, those who are not immune are at risk. Before 20 weeks there is a risk of fetal varicella syndrome with neurological and eye abnormalities. After 36 weeks the fetus can be born with chickenpox. Erythema infectiosum can result in obstetric problems, including hydrops fetalis. The risk is greater in the second trimester.

Pruritic urticarial papules and plaques of pregnancy (PUPPP)

PUPP - rash in pregnancy

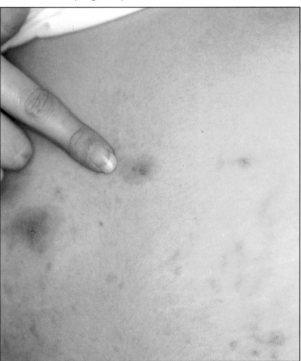

This classically occurs in a primagravida in her 3rd trimester of pregnancy. It starts in abdominal striae, and as the name suggests there are urticarial papules and plaques.

Pemphigoid gestationis

This can occur at anytime in pregnancy. There is a very itchy rash that is initially urticated, that goes on to develop blisters, as in bullous pemphigoid.

Skin and the psyche

The skin reflects our psychological well being. Patients often find their psoriasis relapses at times of stress. They are also anxious about how other people perceive them. Those with alopecia areata frequently have had some major life event before an attack. The child with atopic eczema is constantly scratching and they can develop a detrimental 'itch scratch cycle'. They suffer sleep disturbance and reduced quality of life.

Children can develop localised areas of alopecia from pulling at their hair (trichotillomania). These irregular patches contain broken hairs. Scratching and picking at rashes is common. Some teenagers, usually girls, present with mild acne that is very excoriated and scarred (acne excoriée). Similarly they may have minimal acne but are very incapacitated by it as they have a distorted body image (dysmorphophobia).

Patients with dermatitis artefacta can present with a range of rashes at rather odd sites. One should always consider this possibility when faced with an unusual or unexpected rash. Patients with parasitophobia attend presenting a match box for inspection. This usually contains skin fragments rather than an insect. Sadly they have no insight into their condition and a confrontational approach should be avoided.

Disease states

The patient with diabetes

A patient with diabetes is at increased risk of other metabolic diseases and certain superficial infections. Common dermatological problems are:

- Intertrigo, candida, tinea and boils

- Ulcers

- Necrobiosis lipoidica

- Diffuse granuloma annulare

- Eruptive xanthomas and xanthelasma

The transplant patient

In today's modern age transplants are not uncommon and we are now seeing the survivors who have been on long-term immunosuppressants. These patients are at increased risk of certain infections and malignancies. These include: warts, herpes simplex, herpes zoster, actinic keratoses and squamous cell carcinomas.

Skin problems that can be associated with malignancy

- Acanthosis nigricans

- Generalised pruritus

- Hyperhidrosis

- Dermatomyositis

- Erythema gyratum repens

Common associations with HIV

- Severe seborrhoeic dermatitis

- Oral, hairy leukoplakia

- Giant molluscum contagiosum

- Kaposi's sarcoma

- Pruritus

Emergency dermatology

Dermatological emergencies are uncommon but an important part of primary care. The GP or nurse should know when to ask for help. Airways obstruction can occur with angioedema and anaphylaxis can result from severe peanut and latex allergy. One of the signs of meningococcal meningitis is the purpuric rash.

Erythroderma

This presents as a generalised erythematous rash (more than 90 per cent). Erythroderma can result in loss of temperature control, upset fluid balance, protein loss, anaemia and cardiac failure. It is a dermatological emergency. There can be oedema, lymphadenopathy and loss of nails. The underlying cause may not be obvious and these include the various forms of eczema, psoriasis, pityriasis rubra pilaris, lymphoma and drug eruptions. Exfoliative dermatitis resembles erythroderma, but scaling is more pronounced and requires urgent hospital admission.

Unstable and generalised pustular psoriasis

Psoriasis can become unstable and go on to become erythrodermic. This instability may be precipitated by the sudden cessation of topical steroids. Generalised pustular psoriasis resembles erythroderma but with the addition of sterile pustules.

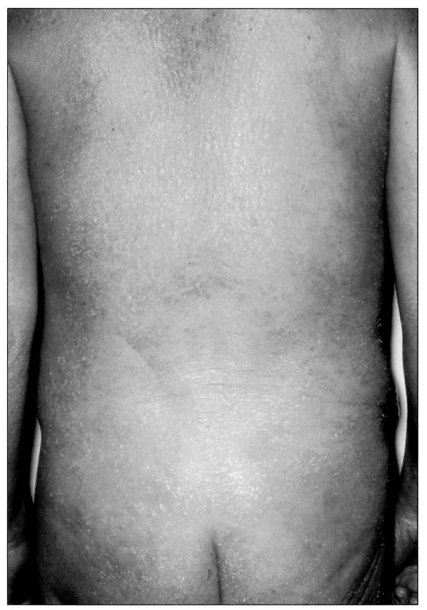

Erythroderma - generalised red rash

Staphylococcal scalded skin syndrome (SSSS)
and
Toxic epidermal necrolysis (TEN)

Staphylococcal scalded skin syndrome is due to infection with a specific phage type of Staph. aureus. The infant presents with blistering, causing loss of skin on a background of erythema. TEN is seen in adults and is usually due to drugs. It produces a similar type of rash.

TEN - toxic epidermal necrolysis

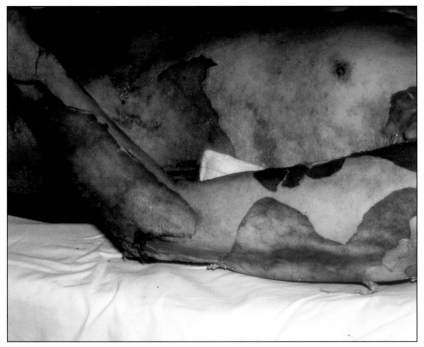

Erysipelas, necrotising fasciitis

Erysipelas is a skin infection produced by streptococci. The patient is often unwell, with a fever, malaise and rash. The face is a common site with a warm, red, oedematous patch. There is distinct demarcation between the normal and abnormal skin and it is worth viewing the rash from different angles.

Erysipelas - note line of demarcation

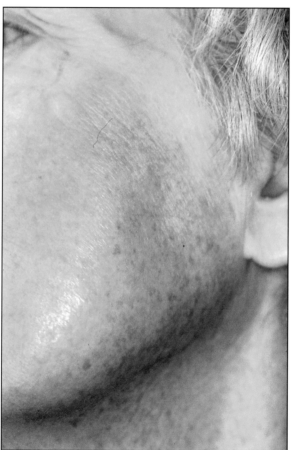

Orbital cellulitis is rare, but needs urgent diagnosis and treatment. It tends to occur in children and be secondary to a minor injury or sinusitis. There is orbital and possibly lid swelling, painful eye movements and a proptosis. A patient with necrotising fasciitis presents with a rapidly expanding, red painful area that undergoes necrosis. This is a dermatological emergency.

Sweet syndrome

The patient presents with a rash, fever and neutrophilia. The rash takes the form of discrete plaques that can contain pustules.

More urgent problems

Some more conditions that can give rise to dermatological emergencies that are covered in other sections of this book:

- Bullous diseases in childhood

- Eczema herpeticum

- Kawasaki disease

- Cellulitis

- Vasculitis

- Pyoderma gangrenosum

Part 5

Lumps

and

bumps

The usual cause for concern is whether a lesion is malignant or not. With any lesion one wants to know when did it appear, and is it solitary? It is useful to know who first noticed the lesion, has it changed and if so over how long?

When examining a lesion it is useful to record the site, size, shape and colour of the lesion. It is worth looking to see if the lesion is symmetrical. Do look for any distortion of the normal skin architecture. It is useful to feel for any induration and remove any crust. The lesion should be inspected in a well lit room and a hand lens should be available.

Benign lesions

Warts

Warts result from a superficial viral infection with the human papilloma virus. The actual appearance of the warts depends on the strain of the virus and the site of the lesion. Developing immunity to a particular strain results in clearing that strains lesions.

Common warts - rough symmetrical lesions

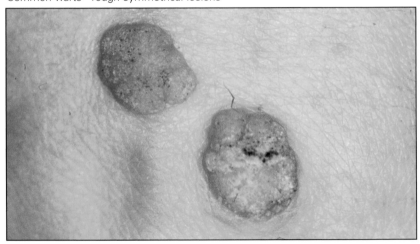

Common warts are frequently found on the backs of children's hands. They appear as rough, symmetrical papules. Plane warts are found on the face and also on the back of the hands. They are tiny flesh coloured or pigmented papules. They can occur in scars (Koebnerisation).

> **Tip:** *A solitary warty lesion in the elderly should be sent for histology to exclude malignancy*

Verruca - note dots within lesion

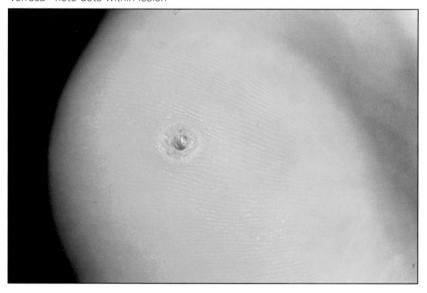

Verrucae are found on the soles of the feet. They are rough lesions covered in callous beneath which are tiny black dots, due to thrombosed capillaries. Verrucae are tender to both direct and lateral pressure. Callosities are tender only to direct pressure and do not have thrombosed capillaries within them. The term mosaic wart is used when grouped warts occur on the feet. Genital warts appear as flesh coloured papules on the penis or vulva.

Molluscum contagiosum

These are due to a pox virus and can occur at any site. Patients with atopic eczema are prone to molluscum and when patients with eczema have molluscum there can be a ring of eczema around the lesions. In HIV there can be extensive and giant lesions.

Molluscum contagiosum - umbilicated papules

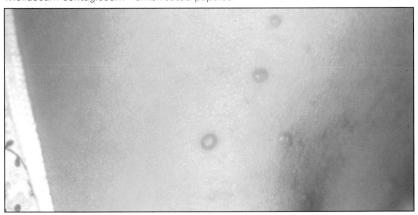

Orf

After exposure to an infected sheep, the individual develops a painful nodule (usually on a digit) that can progress to ulceration.

Orf - ulcerating nodule

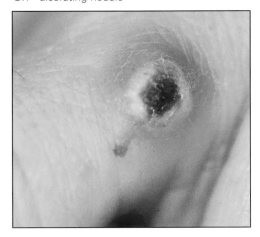

Skin tags (fibroepithelial polyps)

Skin tags are very common. Frequent sites are the neck and axillae. They present as uniform pedunculated flesh coloured papules and nodules.

Seborrhoeic warts (basal cell papillomas – BCP)

These are very common. Their numbers increase with age and sun exposure. Common sites are the forehead and back. The surface is cribriform, waxy and feels greasy. It actually contains plugs of keratin. They have a well-defined edge and have a rather 'stuck on' appearance. Those on the face tend to be flatter and can occasionally be difficult to distinguish from a lentigo maligna. A seborrhoeic wart can be irritated and become inflamed.

Seborrhoeic wart - stuck on appearance

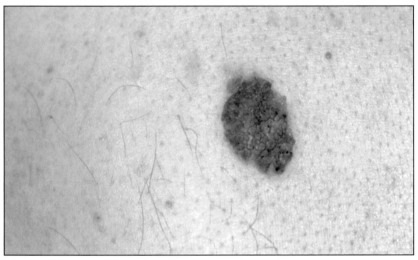

> **Tip:** If a lesion could be an inflamed seborrhoeic wart, try a topical antibiotic for two weeks and review.

Dermatofibroma

This benign lesion can result from an insect bite. They often present as a firm light brown symmetrical nodule on the lower leg. The lesion can be itchy and the surface may be smooth or slightly scaly. There is a peripheral rim of pigmentation and on pinching a dermatofibroma dimples.

Dermatofibroma - usually browner

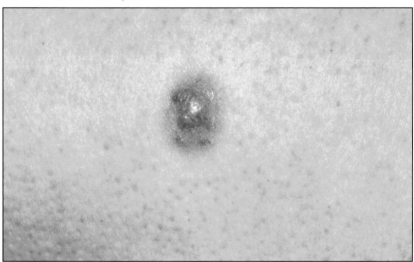

Solar lentiges (liver spots)

These are uniform pigmented patches found on sun exposed sites. The numbers increase with age and sun exposure. The uniformity of pigment and the regularity of the border help distinguish a lentigo, from a lentigo maligna.

Campbell de Morgan spots

These small cherry red papules are found on the trunk and proximal limbs. They are angiomas and appear from middle age onwards.

Pyogenic granuloma

These are benign vascular lesions that probably result from minor trauma. Common sites are the fingers and lips. They appear as a fast growing red pedunculated nodule that bleeds on minimal trauma. They can appear similar to an amelanotic melanoma and a histological diagnosis is required.

Pyogenic granuloma - lesion that bleeds on trauma

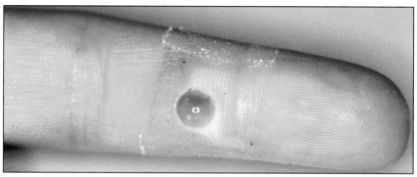

Keloids

These are hypertrophic scars. Keloids present as rather rubbery nodules. Afro-Caribbeans are commonly affected and frequent sites are the shoulders, sternal area and ears.

Keloid - rubbery nodule

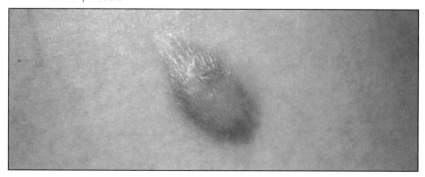

Cysts

There are various cysts that occur in the skin. Most are asymptomatic, unless they become very large or secondarily infected. There are epidermoid cysts (sebaceous cysts) that are derived from the epidermis. These are lined with keratin and have a punctum, through which their contents can be expressed. Pilar cysts are derived from hair follicles and not surprisingly are found on the scalp.

Epidermoid cyst - note punctum

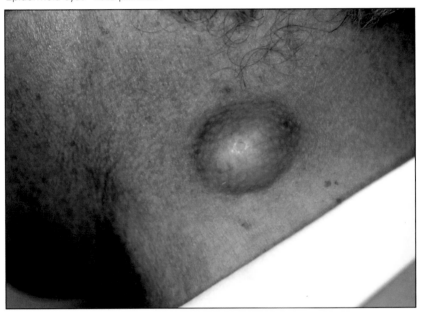

Other benign lesions

Sebaceous gland hyperplasia can occur on the face. They appear as small flesh coloured umbilicated papules that can resemble an early basal cell carcinoma. Senile comedones present as a distended sebaceous gland, with a black core that can be expressed. Calcium can be deposited in the skin as a cutaneous calculus.

Keratoacanthoma

These rapidly expanding tumours are found in the over-50 age group. They are more common in men. There is a rapidly expanding nodule with follicular plug, rather volcano like. Both clinically and histologically they are difficult to distinguish from a squamous cell carcinoma. Although they will resolve if untreated, a keratoacanthoma should be excised and sent for histology to exclude a squamous cell carcinoma.

Keratoacanthoma - volcano-like with keratin plug

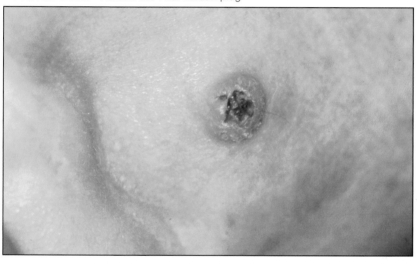

Lipomas

These benign fatty tumours present as slowly enlarging, rubbery, lobulated lesions.

Chondrodermatitis nodularis helices

This presents as a very tender nodule on the external ear. Its extreme tenderness helps distinguish this lesion from an actinic keratosis, or a squamous cell carcinoma. The nodule of chondrodermatitis nodularis is frequently umbilicated, whilst an actinic keratosis is scaly.

Naevi

Banal naevi

Cellular naevus - uniform pigmented papule not enlarging

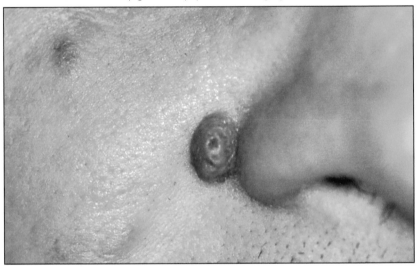

Naevi are either congenital or acquired. However, in practice it is very difficult to tell the difference. The pigment cells in a naevus migrate downwards with age. Hence a junctional naevus can become an intradermal naevus and then a cellular naevus. It is probably easier to call them all banal naevi.

Becker's naevus

First appears in adolescence, often on the shoulder. There is a large pigmented patch with hairs.

Blue naevus

These are found on the limbs and lower back from childhood onwards. They are a deep blue colour. They do not change over time, which helps distinguish them from a melanoma.

Epidermal naevi

These present in childhood. On the trunk and limbs there is a warty linear lesion.

Giant naevus

These large congenital naevi can be quite disfiguring eg the bathing trunk naevus. They do have an increased risk of malignant change.

Spitz naevus

These are found on children's face and limbs. They present as red nodules. They are sometimes known as juvenile melanoma, although this term is misleading as they are a benign lesion.

Halo naevus

Sometimes a naevus develops an area of depigmentation around it. The naevus then resolves and finally the pigmentation returns to normal.

Halo naevi - note rim of depigmentation

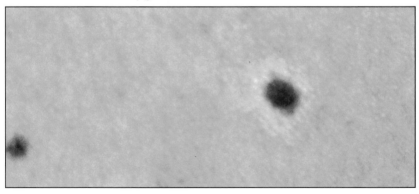

Naevus sebaceous

These naevi are found on the scalp. They are yellow and look rather warty in appearance. In later life basal carcinomas can develop within them.

Skin Cancer

Risk factors for skin cancer

Risk factors for skin cancer include a positive family history, fair skin, blue eyes, and tendency to burn easily and rarely tan on sun exposure, living in sunny climates, being at high altitudes and working outdoors.

Solar radiation contains ultraviolet light 10 per cent, visible light 50 per cent and infrared light 40 per cent. Ultraviolet light can be further divided into UVC, UVB and UVA. The ozone layer filters out the UVC. Traditionally UVA was thought to cause ageing and the UVB burning and cancer. However, increasingly both UVB and UVA are being implicated in skin cancer. The UV light is absorbed by the cells resulting in cellular and molecular damage. Then incomplete and incorrect repair of the DNA leads to development of malignancy. Sunburn in childhood is implicated in melanoma and long term sun exposure in non melanoma skin cancer.

Patients with vitiligo are at increased risk of skin cancer. Skin cancers can develop in scars from injuries, burns and after exposure to radiation. The ingestion of arsenic and taking immunosuppressive medication increases the risk of certain skin cancers. There are syndromes in which skin cancers occur, although these are quite rare and sun exposure is quite common.

Referral for diagnosis

Do make use of local guidelines and pathways of care for the diagnosis of skin cancer. Do make use of fast track and pigmented lesion clinics. However, do not clog up the system with obvious seborrhoeic warts.

Basal cell carcinoma (BCC) rodent ulcer

Basal cell carcinomas are found on exposed sites such as the head, neck and chest, but surprisingly spare the hands. Basal cell carcinomas are slow growing and rarely metastasise. They can present as a cystic lesion

Nodular BCC

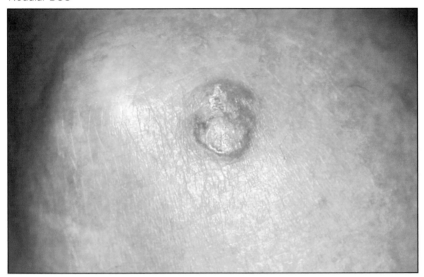

Pigmented BCC

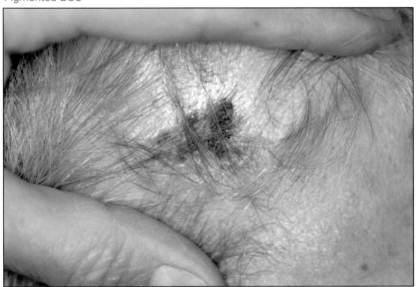

Superficial BCC

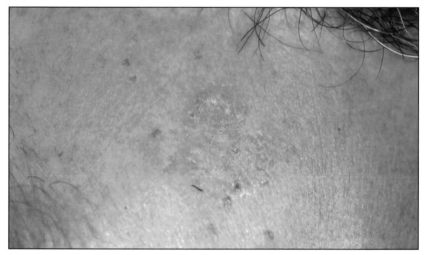

or as a nodule. They have a pearly translucent appearance with telangiectasia and can go on to ulcerate. Basal cell carcinomas can be pigmented and then need to be differentiated from a malignant melanoma.

Basal cell carcinoma may appear as a superficial plaque with a pearly rolled edge and stretching this border makes it more obvious. A morphoeic or sclerosing lesion presents as a yellow patch similar to scar tissue. This can resemble eczema, or a patch of Bowen's disease.

Tip: *Stretching a BCC makes the edge more obvious.*

Patients with Gorlin's Syndrome have multiple basal cell carcinomas and palmar and plantar pits. This syndrome is inherited as an autosomal dominant. There are also cysts in the jaw, other skeletal abnormalities and ectopic calcification.

Actinic keratoses (AK), (solar keratosis)

These are extremely common. They present as rough raised scaly lesion on sun exposed sites. They can be red or flesh coloured. Common sites are the bald head, face, ears and backs of hands. They are usually multiple and easily felt. They vary in size between 1mm to 1 cm. These lesions rarely progress to a squamous cell carcinoma. Induration of the base of the lesion would suggest the lesion could have progressed to a squamous cell carcinoma.

Actinic keratosis - rough superficial lesions

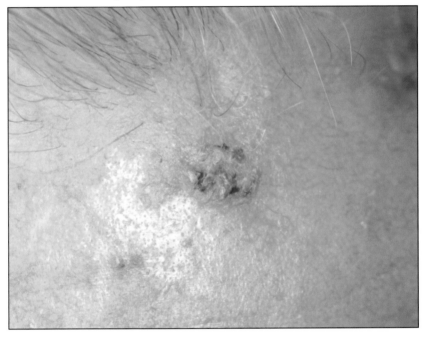

Tip: The bald male scalp is a favourite site for actinic keratoses.

Bowen's disease

This is a form of carcinoma in situ. The lower legs is favourite site. Bowen's presents as red, scaly, patches on sun exposed areas. There can be a little crusting and induration. This can progress to a frank squamous cell carcinoma. The differential diagnosis includes psoriasis and actinic keratoses.

Bowens disease - red scaly patch

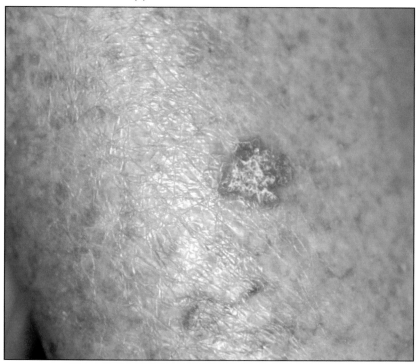

> **Tip:** If a patient has a solitary patch of 'psoriasis' do consider if it could be Bowen's disease.

Squamous cell carcinoma (SCC) (epithelioma)

These malignant tumours occur on sun exposed sites. They can develop from AKs, in Bowen's disease and from chronic ulcers. Patients on immunosuppressives are at greatly increased risk. Favoured sites are the face, scalp, ears and backs of hands. Those on the lip and ear tend to behave more aggressively.

Squamous cell carcinoma

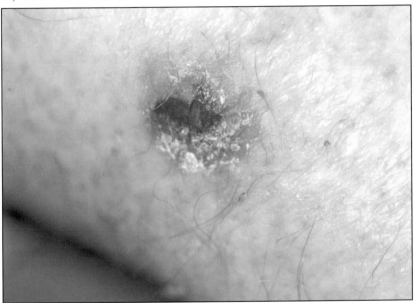

Squamous cell carcinomas presents as a fleshy nodule, or crusted lesion that can ulcerate. They are indurated and have a craggy edge. One should be suspicious of a slowly growing non-healing ulcer.

> **Tip:** The normal skin surface and markings are lost over a squamous cell carcinoma.

Melanoma

Melanoma is so important because the outlook for patients diagnosed with thin lesions is good, whilst the prognosis for patients with thick lesions is very poor. Melanoma is associated with excessive sun exposure, especially sun burn at an early age. Those with fair skin and a tendency to burn are at increased risk. Those who have had one melanoma are at increased risk of another. Other risk factors are having a positive history of melanoma, the presence of atypical, giant, or multiple benign naevi.

Atypical (dysplastic naevi) have variegated pigmentation and an irregular border. They are often multiple. They are a risk factor for melanoma and any rapid change in size, shape, or colour would be a prompt for an excision biopsy.

Superficial spreading melanoma - beware the changing lesion!

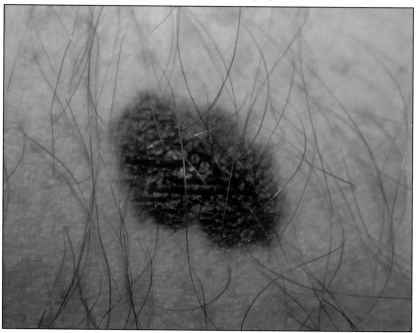

Superficial spreading melanoma

The superficial spreading melanoma is more common on the lower legs of females. The nodular lesion is more common on the backs of males. Patients are becoming more aware of melanoma and the need for early consultation. However males tend to be less likely to consult than females. The superficial melanoma presents as a macule or patch that has recently changed in size, shape or colour. Approximately 50 per cent of melanomas arise from previous benign moles and 50 per cent as a new lesion.

Superficial spreading melanoma - note asymmetry

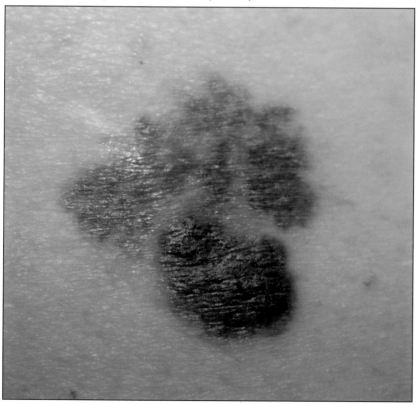

Superficial spreading melanoma check lists

There are various check lists for melanoma. The A, B, C, D, E checklist:

A Asymmetry

B Border (irregularity)

C Colour variation

D Diameter

E Enlargement (recent)

Or has the pigmented lesion recently:

- Changed in size

- Changed in colour

- Developed an irregular outline

- Has it mixed colour

- Ulceration

- Any inflammation

- Bleeding, crusting, inflammation

Excision biopsy of a suspicious pigmented lesion is the gold standard. Photography and follow up may be of value in low risk cases. The dermatoscope can be useful in experienced hands.

> **Tip:** The normal skin surface and markings are lost over a squamous cell carcinoma.

Nodular melanoma

Nodular melanoma - black nodule

One cannot rely on checklists alone as they are only a guide. A nodular melanoma can be symmetrical and can be only a single colour. It may present as a deep black lesion. It may present as a nodule in an existing mole or as a nodule in a lentigo maligna. Secondary deposits present as black rubbery

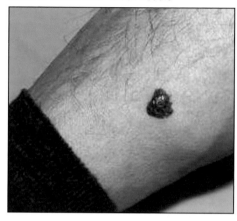

Nodular melanoma - black nodule

lesions. The lymph nodes can be involved, along with secondary deposits in the liver, lung and brain.

Lentigo maligna

Lentigo maligna - note irregular border

These tend to present in older patients, they present as either a pigmented macule or patch on the face. This lesion can be pale brown to black in colour. It increases in size and shows variation in pigment. There is an irregular border. A lentigo maligna needs to be differentiated from a seborrhoeic wart, which

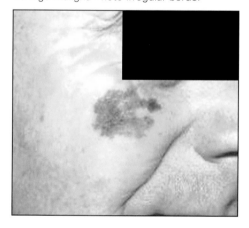

Lentigo maligna - note irregular border

on the face do not tend to be as raised as on the trunk. A lentigo maligna can go on to develop a nodule with it. If a lentigo maligna has been treated with cryotherapy, then this nodule may be amelanotic.

Amelanotic melanoma

An amelanotic melanoma can present as a red nodule. Any presumed pyogenic granuloma is better in a pot, than on the skin, as it should go for histology to exclude an amelanotic melanoma.

Acral melanoma

These are found on the palms and soles near and under nails. Pigmentation extending onto the nail fold in a Caucasian patient is suspicious, but not diagnostic of a melanoma.

> *Tip:* *Refer pigmented lesions rather than doing incisional biopsies.*

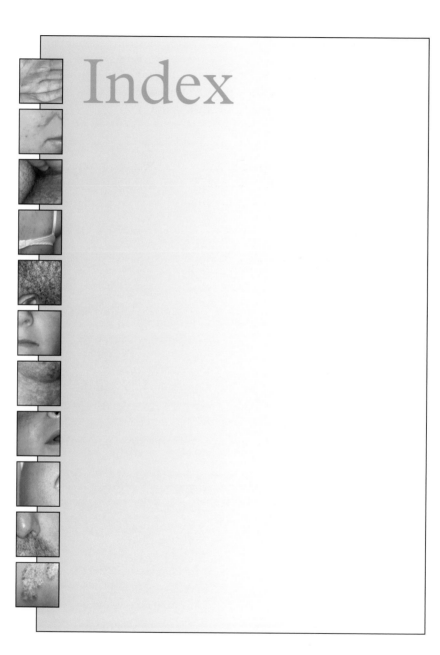

Index

Appendix I
Useful
websites

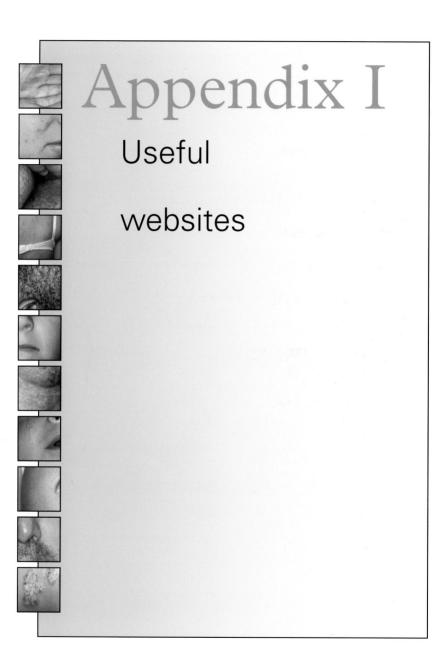

Useful websites

Primary Care Dermatology Society

www.pcds.org.uk

The British Association of Dermatologists

www.bad.org.uk/about/

British Dermatology Nursing Group

www.bdng.org.uk/

American Academy of Dermatology

www.aad.org/

New Zealand Dermatological Society

www.dermnetnz.org/

Cardiff University Department of Dermatology

www.dermatology.org.uk/

Skin Care Campaign

www.skincarecampaign.org

Department of Health:
Guidelines for urgent referral of patients with suspected cancer

www.nice.org.uk

Appendix II

What's likely

from the

signs and

symptoms?

Picking up on major symptom or signs can be very useful. Is the rash itchy and, if so, how severe and for how long? Don't forget family history and medications. On examination do look at the site, colour, distribution and morphology of the rash. One should also look at the size and shape of the individual lesions. The surface of the rash, especially the presence or absence of scale is very important.

Itchy rashes

Very itchy

Lichen planus

Scabies

Urticaria and dermatographism

Lichen simplex

Dermatitis herpetiformis

Nodular prurigo

Mycosis fungoides

Actinic prurigo

Itchy

Eczema / dermatitis (various types)

Tinea pedis

Pediculosis capitis

Polymorphic light eruption

Variable itch

Psoriasis

Pityriasis rosea

Itch but little rash

Anaemia, polycythaemia

Liver disease, renal disease

Thyroid disease, diabetes

Scaly rashes

Eczema / dermatitis
(various types)

Psoriasis (silvery scale)

Lichen planus

Tinea (various sites)

Pityriasis rosea (scale just inside the edge of the lesions)

Pityriasis versicolor (fine scale)

Pityriasis lichenoides chronica
(scale can be picked off in one piece)

Pityriasis rubra pilaris
(islands of normal skin)

Eczemas / dermatitis

Acute eczema / dermatitis

Erythema

Exudates

Blistering

Chronic eczema / dermatitis

Scaly

Dry

Lichenification

Fissures

What's likely from the signs and symptoms

Infected
eczema / dermatitis

Pathogen – Staph. aureus

Weeping

Pustulation

Impetiginized

Rapid deterioration

Types of eczemas / dermatitis
Atopic
eczema / dermatitis

Atopy – asthma, eczema
and hay fever

In front of elbows and behind knees

Red, itchy, scaly rash

Background dry skin

Allergic contact
eczema / dermatitis

Nickel, chromate, perfumes

Topical medications

Eczema at site of contact

Patch test to confirm

Irritant contact
eczema / dermatitis

Common site – hands

Weak irritants – water and soap

Strong irritants – petrol and acids

Occupations – wet work
and solvents

Seborrhoeic
eczema / dermatitis

Face – nasolabial folds

Scalp – greasy scaly rash

Chest – petaloid lesions

Flexures – infected scaly rash

Discoid eczema

Very itchy rash

Coin shaped lesions

Covered in a crust

Often infected

Pompholyx

Hands and feet

Itchy rash

Vesicles and blisters

Asteatotic eczema

Elderly

Legs

Dry skin

Crazy paving appearance

Stasis eczema

Lower legs

Eczematous rash

Venous disease

Lichen simplex

Itchy, scaly patches

Well defined

Increased markings

Papulosquamous rashes
Rashes with scaly lesions with a well defined margin

Psoriasis

Lichen planus

Reiter's syndrome

Chronic superficial dermatitis

Drug eruptions

Psoriasis

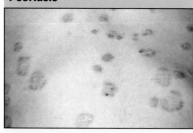

Elbows, knees, lower back

Well defined plaques

Silvery scale

Nail involvement

Lichen planus

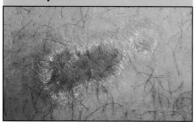

Limbs

Mouth, scalp

Very itchy rash

Lichen planus - continued

Red-mauve scaly papules

Staining of the skin

Nail involvement

Tinea

Itchy scaly rash

Raised border

Confirm by mycology

Pustular rashes

Acne

Rosacea

Pustular psoriasis
(local and generalised)

Folliculitis

Blistering rashes

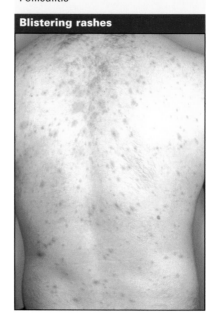

Blistering rashes - continued

Insect bites

Solar reactions

Acute eczemas eg pompholyx

Herpetic lesions
(usually vesicles)

Varicella infections

Pemphigus
(bullae easily rupture)

Pemphigoid

Dermatitis herpetiformis (vesicles)

Porphyrias

Bullous erythema multiforme

Drugs

Scarring rashes

Severe acne

Discoid lupus – common site face

Porphyria cutanea tarda – face
and dorsum of hands

Xeroderma pigmentosa

Immunobullous disease

Rashes often improved by sunlight

Acne

Psoriasis
(10 per cent aggravated)

Seborrhoeic dermatitis

Rashes that 'don't like' sunlight

Actinic prurigo

Juvenile spring eruption

Polymorphic light eruption

Solar urticaria

Actinic reticuloid

DLE and SLE

Phorphyrias

Darier's disease

Drug-related photosensitivity

Morphology of drug rashes

Urticarial

Toxic erythema

Lichenoid

Bullous

Fixed drug eruption

Scalps

Alopecia localised

Scaling – tinea capitis

Scarring – discoid lupus
erythematosus, lichen planus

Normal surface – alopecia areata

Alopecia generalised

Iron deficiency

Thyroid disease

SLE

Syphilis

What's likely from the signs and symptoms

Scaly scalps

Seborrhoeic eczema

Psoriasis

Tinea Capitis

Localised patches

Lichen simplex

Morphoea & lichen sclerosus

Bowen's disease

Tinea corporis

Granuloma annulare

Koebner phenomenon

Psoriasis

Lichen planus

Sarcoid

Plane warts

Increased pigmentation

Freckle

Lentigo

Chloasma and melasma

Post-inflammatory
hyperpigmentation

Decreased pigmentation

Vitiligo

Post inflammatory
hypopigmentation

Pityriasis alba (cheeks)

Lichen sclerosus et atrophicus

Leprosy

Vascular disease

Spider naevi

Common in pregnancy

Often on face

Blanch on pressure

Rashes with telangiectasia

Hereditary

Pregnancy, liver disease

Rashes induced by topical
steroids

SLE, dermatomyositis

Lichen sclerosus

Rashes on the hands

Eczema
(atopy, contact, pompholyx)

Psoriasis
(plaque, localised pustular)

Lichen planus

Scabies

Granuloma annulare

Vitiligo

Rashes on feet

Eczema

Psoriasis
(plaque, localised)

Tinea pedis

Juvenile plantar dermatosis

Pitted keratolysis

Malignant lesions

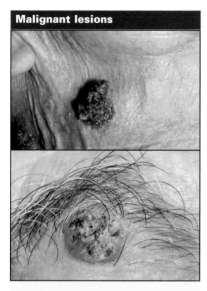

Basal cell carcinoma

Squamous cell carcinoma
(see illustrations above)

Bowen's disease
(intraepidermal carcinoma)

Melanoma

Types of basal cell carcinoma

Cystic

Nodular

Superficial

Morphoeic (sclerosing)

Pigmented

Types of melanoma

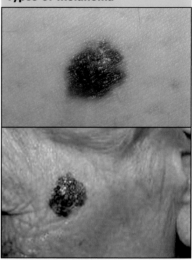

Superficial spreading
(see upper illustration)

Nodular

Lentigo maligna
(see lower illustration)

Acral melanoma

Amelanotic melanoma

What's likely from the signs and symptoms

Nail changes

Psoriasis

Onychomycosis

Trauma

Lichen planus

Alopecia areata

Tumour

Ulceration

Arterial

Venous

Diabetic (neuropathic)

Malignant

Pyoderma gangrenosum

Artefacta

Rheumatoid arthritis

Sickle cell disease

Arterial ulcer

Painful

Foot or shin

Punched out

Reduced or absent
peripheral pulses

Venous ulcer

Lower leg

Superficial, larger than arterial

Oedema, hyperpigmentation

Eczema

Varicose veins

Diabetic ulcers

Over bony prominences

Deep

Painless

Covered in callous

Lesions
(see lumps and bumps)

Benign skin lesions

Viral warts

Molluscum contagiosum

Seborrhoeic warts

Dermatofibroma

Pyogenic granuloma
(exclude amelanotic melanoma)

Keratoacanthoma
(exclude SCC)

Actinic keratoses
(low risk of malignant change)

Viral warts

Common

Verruca

Mosaic

Plane

Filiform

Genital